SHAMAN,

HEALER,

SAGE

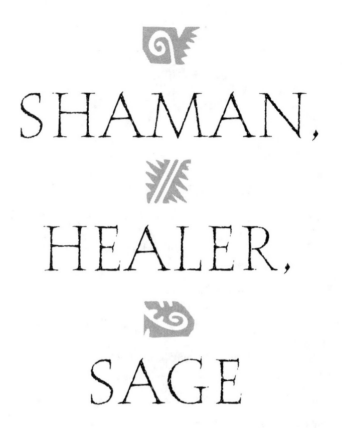

SHAMAN,

HEALER,

SAGE

How to Heal Yourself and Others with the Energy Medicine of the Americas

ALBERTO VILLOLDO, PH.D.

HARMONY BOOKS
NEW YORK

Published by Harmony Books, New York, New York.
Member of the Crown Publishing Group.
Random House, Inc. New York, Toronto, London, Sydney, Auckland
www.randomhouse.com
Harmony Books is a registered trademark and the Harmony Books colophon is a trademark of Random House, Inc.

Printed in the United States of America

Design by Lauren Dong

Illustrations by Nicole Kaufman

Library of Congress Cataloging-in-Publication Data
Villoldo, Alberto.
    Shaman, healer, sage : how to heal yourself and others with the energy medicine of the Americas / by Alberto Villoldo.—1st ed.
    Includes index.
        1. Shamanism—South America.   2. Mental healing.   I. Title.
    BF1622.S63 V55   2000
    299'.833—dc21
                                                        00-035010
    ISBN 0-609-60544-5

10 9 8

To my mother Elena, with all my love

ACKNOWLEDGMENTS

THERE ARE NO WORDS THAT CAN EXPRESS MY GRATITUDE TO THE PER-sons who made this book possible. First and foremost is my mentor, Don Antonio, who had the patience, vision, and endurance to train a young Western anthropologist in the shamanic arts. My editor, Patty Gift at Random House, has immersed herself in the medicine teachings, accompanying me to the highest mountains of the Andes to work with the last Inka elders. I owe her my immeasurable grati-tude for making this book a reality. My heartfelt thanks to Laura Wood and Normandi Ellis, for helping shape the manuscript; to Stanley Krippner, for believing in me and supporting my research during my early years; and to my agent, Sue Berger, for her steadfast encouragement. Last, I want to acknowledge the contributions made by the students and faculty of the Healing the Light Body School in shaping the techniques and practices discussed herein, and Lisa Summerlot, for her untiring love and support.

CONTENTS

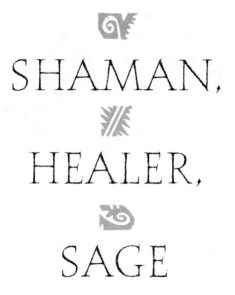

SHAMAN,

HEALER,

SAGE

PROLOGUE

THIS BOOK IS THE RESULT OF MY TRAVELS AND TRAINING WITH THE Inka shamans. One of the great civilizations of the Americas and the builders of Machu Picchu, the Inka lived in cities in the clouds with cobblestone streets that were cleaned every night by releases of water from the city's canal system. Inka shamans practiced energy medicine for more than five thousand years, transmitting this knowledge from one generation to the next through an oral tradition. For twenty-five years I studied with the finest Inka medicine men and women. The rites I underwent in the high mountains of the Andes and the Amazon adhered to ancient tradition and sometimes required months of preparation. They freed the apprentice from living in the grip of fear, greed, violence, and predatory sexuality. My quest was guided by an old Inka named Antonio Morales. My adventures in the Amazon and the Andean highlands with Don Antonio are documented in my earlier books, *Dance of the Four Winds* and *Island of the Sun.*

The techniques for healing with spirit and light in this book are my contemporary reinterpretation of ancient healing practices. Versions of the shaman's way of seeing that I call the Second Awareness and the Extraction Process are still in use in North and South America. The Death Rites originate in the Amazon and form part of a body of knowledge discovered by men and women who have transcended our notions of time and death. The Illumination Process I developed with my mentor Don Antonio from the remnants of a nearly forgotten Inka practice for healing through the Luminous Energy Field. These techniques are extraordinarily powerful and effective. They must be used only with the strongest code of ethics and integrity.

Part I provides a background of the belief system on which these techniques are based. Part II provides techniques for learning the shaman's way of seeing and for creating sacred space and practices you can experiment with for your personal healing. Please do not use them with others without adequate training from a master practitioner. Part III describes advanced techniques that must be performed by a master practitioner, a person who has undergone an apprenticeship overseen by a skilled teacher. These chapters describe procedures used for unblocking the immune response, for extracting intrusive energies and entities, as well as assisting a loved one who is making his or her return journey to the Spirit world.

There are dangers associated with energy healing, both for the client and for the healer. Far too many poorly trained practitioners dispense energy healing without understanding the mechanics of the human energy field. I have seen people diagnosed with cancer receive "energy healing" on their tumor, only to have the cancer spread throughout their body. To their disbelief, they discovered that cancer thrives on certain forms of energy. I have also seen persons suffering from serious psychological conditions who have been treated by unqualified healers, only to have their conditions exacerbated and the symptoms of their neuroses or their dysfunctional worldview reinforced. In one case, a woman came to see me after losing her child in an automobile accident. She had been to a psychic who said that her little girl was always by her side, that all she had to do was to "be open" and she would feel the presence of her daughter. The woman felt an immediate sense of relief. Yet after a few days she began to suffer from insomnia. After a week of no sleep she came to see me. The first thing she said was that she wanted to die and was ready to take her own life. When I tested her for the presence of an intrusive entity (see Chapter 8), I discovered she tested positive. The girl's spirit had attached itself to her mother's Luminous Energy Field, seeking refuge from the confusion and agitation one experiences after a traumatic death. The healer's advice to "be open," although well intended, was keeping both mother and daughter in emotional turmoil and psychic pain.

In our first session the mother released her daughter to the luminous healers who would carry her to the light of the Spirit world. It was difficult for her to let go. During the Illumination Process she saw death as a doorway to infinity; she experienced that her daughter was separated from her only by a thin veil. Shortly thereafter she began sleeping soundly again. We then sealed the opening in her Luminous Energy Field through which the girl's spirit had entered. Like an open wound, this tear in her energy field was an invitation to opportunistic spirit entities and disturbing energies. We then spent the next few sessions healing her grief. I encouraged her to go to a psychotherapist who specialized in treating persons recovering from loss. I'm convinced that the mother would have committed suicide had she continued to follow the psychic's advice. Instead, she engaged her healing journey with courage and dedication. Today she is a gifted and compassionate healer, assisting others who have suffered loss and bereavement in their lives.

BLACK AND WHITE MAGIC

When I was in my early twenties, I was preparing for an expedition to the Amazon when I received a call from the foundation that sponsored my research. They needed an anthropologist to complete a study on Voodoo healers in Haiti. I was reluctant to go, as I knew very little of the African-derived healing practices in Haiti. The foundation officer explained that it would be for only ten days, to assist the senior anthropologist on the project, and persuaded me when he mentioned he was reviewing my grant application to return to the Amazon. Five days later I landed in Port-au-Prince. The senior anthropologist was a man in his late thirties who had spent the better part of a year in Haiti. He explained to me that the French who colonized the island had been the worst slave drivers in the New World.

Whereas the average life expectancy of an African slave after he arrived in America was thirty years, the life expectancy of a slave who had the misfortune of landing in Haiti was only two years. He went on to explain that Voodoo was originally a healing practice from sub-Saharan Africa, and that in Haiti it was also used to harm one's foes, particularly the ruthless slave masters. The techniques were identical, he explained. The same practices you used to heal someone could be used to hurt someone. The same techniques that were used to stimulate the immune system to eradicate a cancerous tumor could be used to lay waste to the immune system so that your victim would die from pneumonia in a matter of weeks.

Being in my early twenties, I was convinced that I knew better. Black magic, I conjectured, could work only on those who believed in it. If you did not subscribe to the belief system, it could not affect you. I remember stating this matter-of-factly to the senior anthropologist as we sat at a small café by the waterfront. He looked at me and smiled. "I'm willing to put my money on that," I said. "Done," he replied. We agreed on a hundred-dollar wager that Voodoo could not affect me. We headed off to the home of the Voodoo priest he had been working with. The old man lived in a ramshackle wooden hut on a hilltop overlooking the town. After casual introductions in the local Haitian Creole, which my colleague spoke fluently, he proceeded to explain to the man that I was a nonbeliever, that I thought the old man's magic was all make-believe, and that he wanted to teach me a lesson. I understood enough French to pick up some of the words. "Don't hurt him," he said. The old man turned to me and smiled. "You want believe?" he asked in broken English, and laughed loudly. We agreed that he would do his work on Monday of the following week, after I returned to California.

On the appointed day I was having dinner with friends, telling them about my Haiti experience and the healing power of Voodoo. I was pontificating on how belief was an important ingredient in the equation, both for healing the sick or harming adversaries. If you lived outside the belief system, I explained, it simply did not work, and I was living proof, as that very evening the meanest Voodoo priest in Haiti was working on me, to no avail. Everyone raised his or her glass of wine to my health. That was Monday evening. On Tuesday and Wednesday I felt fine, but come Thursday midafternoon I developed a headache that by early evening had turned into a migraine. By eight o'clock my gut had twisted into a knot, I was having intestinal spasms, and I was retching uncontrollably. At midnight the phone rang with a collect call from the anthropologist in Haiti. They had been unable to work on me on Monday, as we had agreed, but had done so that day. He had just returned to his hotel from the ceremony and wanted to know if I felt anything. I groaned into the phone and told him to go back to the Voodoo priest and ask him to undo whatever it was he had done. At that point, even death would have been a welcome relief.

By the following morning I was nearly recovered and managed to convince myself that I had picked up some intestinal bug. I went to the university health center, where my doctor ran tests and found that I was clear of any parasites. The lesson cost me a hundred dollars, which at that time was a lot of money for a graduate student, and one of the worst nights of my life. I discovered that just as you can help people through energy healing, you can also hurt them. I would later learn that energy healing from a poorly trained practitioner is often tantamount to black magic, regardless of how well-meaning the healer is. Black magic happens not only in Haiti and the bayous of Louisiana but anywhere well-meaning but poorly trained individuals lay their hands on others, attempting to perform healing, and unknowingly transmit toxic energy to them. Students will sometimes comment that this can't happen if you are sending love to another person, as this energy is supposedly pure and holy. I remind these students of the pain that we can inflict on others in the name of love. In time, I discovered another kind of black magic we do to ourselves: the negative thoughts and beliefs that keep us from our personal power and wreak havoc on our immune system.

The most important lesson for me that night, though, was the crucial role of the healer's ethics and intent. Much of the shaman's decade-long training is dedicated to developing a high ethic, a value system founded on a deep reverence for all life. Only then can the techniques be properly mastered. Similarly, a doctor of Western medicine spends at least five years learning his or her craft. Is it prudent to turn my health care over to someone who has taken a weekend workshop in energy medicine?

This is the quandary for Westerners who take a short training in energy medicine or shamanism. If you have a calling to practice energy medicine, take the time to train with teachers whose integrity, wisdom, and technical knowledge will assist you to develop your own spiritual gifts.

My own journey into shamanism was guided by my desire to become whole. In healing my own soul wounds, I learned to love myself and others. I walked the path of the wounded healer and learned to transform the pain, grief, anger, and shame that lived within me into sources of strength and compassion. I was able to feel for another's pain because I knew what it was like to hurt. In the Healing the Light Body School every student embarks on a journey of self-healing in which he or she transforms soul wounds into sources of power. Students learn that this is one of the greatest gifts that they will later offer to their clients: the opportunity to discover the power within pain. Students also learn that healing is a journey their client embarks upon, not a procedure the healer performs.

Last, I want to state that the healing methods in this book are my own synthesis and interpretation of ancient healing practices. I do not speak for my teachers, for the Inka, or for Native American shamans. Although I had the privilege of training with the finest Inka medicine people, I make no claim to be presenting a body of Inka traditions. The healing practices described herein are what I learned in my training as a shaman, and I take full responsibility for their beauty and their shortcomings.

PART I

TEACHINGS

OF THE

SHAMANS

Native American shamans have practiced energy medicine for more than five thousand years. Some medicine people believe their spiritual lineage extends back even further. They remember stories handed down from grandmother to granddaughter that speak about when the Earth was young. Even though the Americas' early inhabitants had a complex astronomical knowledge, advanced mathematics, and sophisticated architecture, writing never developed in the Americas as it did elsewhere. Scholars overlooked the Native American spiritual traditions in favor of Judaism, Christianity, and Buddhism, which left behind written records. For example, while Western theologians have been studying Buddhism for more than two centuries, it has been only in the last forty years that any serious interest has emerged in the study of Native American spirituality. The study of shamanism was left to anthropologists, who, with notable exceptions such as Margaret Mead, were poorly trained to study the spirit.

The wholesale destruction of the North American Indians by the European settlers drove the remaining Native Americans into disease-ridden reservations, where the elders carefully guarded the spiritual traditions. Understandably, the elders grew reluctant to share their heritage with the white dominators. The Indios in Peru fared no better. The Spanish conquistadors came to Peru seeking gold and therefore left the Inka spiritual traditions largely undisturbed. Yet what the conquistadors overlooked, the missionaries sought to obliterate.

The scraggly band of gold seekers that arrived on the South American continent brought a set of beliefs that were incomprehensible to the Indios. The first was that all of the food of the world belonged by divine right to humans—specifically the Europeans—who were masters over the animals and plants of the Earth. The second belief was that humans could not speak to the rivers, to the animals, to the mountains, or to God. And the third was that humankind had to wait until the end of all time before tasting infinity.

Nothing could have seemed more absurd to the Native Americans. While the Europeans believed they had been cast out of the mythical Garden of Eden, the Indios understood they were the stewards and caretakers of the Garden. They still spoke with the thundering rivers and the whispering mountains and still heard the voice of God in the wind. The Spanish chroniclers in Peru wrote that when the conquistador Pizarro met the Inka ruler Atahualpa, he handed him the Bible, explaining to him that this was the word of God. The Inka brought the volume to his ear, listened carefully for a few moments, and then threw the holy book to the ground, exclaiming, "What kind of god is this that does not speak?"

In addition to the silence of the European God, the Native Americans were confounded by His gender. The conquistadors brought with them a patriarchal mythology that intimidated the Native American feminine traditions. Before the arrival of the Spanish, Mother Earth and her feminine forms—the caves, lagoons, and other openings into the earth—represented the divine principles. The Europeans imposed the masculine divine principle—the phallus, or tree of life. Church steeples rose to heaven. The feminine Earth was no longer worshiped or respected. The trees, animals, and forests were available for plundering.

Today we still live in the grip of this disconnected worldview. We believe that if it does not breathe, move, or grow, it is not alive. We view energy from sources such as wood, oil, or coal as a fuel that we employ. In the ancient world, energy was considered the living fabric of the Universe. Energy was creation made manifest. Perhaps the most important contemporary expression of this belief was formulated by Albert Einstein when he described the relationship between energy and matter in his equation $E = MC^2$. In the West we identify with the side of matter, which is by nature finite. The shaman identifies with the side of energy, which is by nature infinite.

There is another fundamental difference between the ancient Americans and the modern ones. Today we are people of the precept. We are a rule-driven society that relies on documents such as the Constitution, the Ten Commandments, or laws passed by elected officials to bring order to our lives. We change precepts (rules or laws) when we want to change the world. The ancient Greeks, on the other hand, were people of the concept. They were interested not in rules but rather in ideas. They believed that a single idea could change the world and that there was nothing as powerful as an idea whose time had come. Shamans are people of the percept. When they want to change the world, they engage in perceptual shifts that change their relationship to life. They envision the possible, and the outer world changes. This is why a group of Inka elders will sit in meditation envisioning the kind of world they want their grandchildren to inherit.

One reason why the practices of energy healing have been kept so closely guarded is that they are often mistaken for a set of techniques, in the same way that Western medicine is sometimes regarded as a set of procedures. We mistakenly think that we can master energy healing by learning the rules. However, for the shaman it is not about the rules or ideas. It's about vision and Spirit. And while the healing practices often vary from village to village, the Spirit never varies. True healing is nothing less than an awakening to a vision of our healed nature and the experience of infinity.

CHAPTER 1

HEALING AND INFINITY

We have been walking for days. I told Antonio that I did not mind paying for us to take a bus or even a taxi. But he would have nothing to do with it. Would not even let me hire horses. "My people have always walked," he said. And he loves to point out how he can outwalk me even though he is nearly seventy.

Took my shoes off when we arrived at Sillustani, and soaked my feet in the icy lake. This is an eerie place, a cemetery extending over dozens of miles, like the Valley of the Kings in Egypt. Only shamans, kings, and queens are buried here, in gigantic stone towers at the edge of Lake Titicaca. The finest stonemasons came from this land. How did this technology develop here, at the lake on top of the world?

Antonio explained that the burial towers, or chulpas, not only commemorate the dead shamans but also are their temporary homes when they return to visit our world. They are completely liberated, powerful spirits who could materialize whenever they wished. This didn't make me feel any more at ease. We had come here to spend the night, to do ceremony to honor these ancient shamans.

"They've stepped outside of time," he said. He explained that if my faith in reality was based on the belief that time runs in one direction only, then I will be shattered by an experience of my future. "It takes great skill to taste the future and not allow your knowledge to spoil your actions or the present."

JOURNALS

I ENTERED A CAREER IN PSYCHOLOGY AND, LATER, MEDICAL ANTHRO-
pology with a fascination for the human mind. In the 1980s I spent
hundreds of hours in anatomy laboratories. I wanted to know how the
mind could influence the body to create either health or disease. At
that time I had little interest in spirituality, whether of the traditional
or New Age variety. I was convinced that science was the only reliable
method for acquiring knowledge. One day at the University of California I was slicing brain tissue, preparing slides to examine under the
microscope. The brain is the most bewildering organ in the body. Its
crevasses make it resemble a three-pound walnut. These valleys and
convolutions were the only way nature could accommodate a thin
but extensive layer of neocortex (the word means "new brain") into
our heads without increasing the size of our skull. Human evolution
had already run into an anatomically insurmountable obstacle in its
search for a more intelligent brain: The pelvic girdle could not tolerate passing a larger head through the birth canal.

Under the microscope one can observe the millions of synapses
that weave every brain cell with its neighbors in an extraordinary network of living fibers. These neural networks transmit vast amounts of
motor and sensory data. Yet the fascination with the brain is uniquely
Western. The Egyptians had very little use for it, liquefying it after
death and siphoning it off, even though the rest of the body's organs
were mummified. The question we had been debating that day at the
lab was whether the human mind was confined to the brain, or even
to the body, for that matter. I knew that if the brain were simple
enough for us to understand it, *we* would be so simple that we
couldn't. Yet no matter how meticulously we examined slides of the
brain, the mind kept eluding us. The more I learned about the brain,
the more confounded I became about the mind.

I believed that the human race had managed to survive for a million years before the arrival of modern medicine because the body-mind knew the pathways to health. We survived cuts that became infected, and bones broken from falling down a ravine on the way to the watering hole. Until fifty years ago, going to a doctor was more dangerous to your health than staying home and letting your body-mind take its own course. By the early part of the twentieth century, medicine excelled only in the area of diagnosis. It still lacked the curative techniques, effective drugs, and surgical interventions that would not be developed until around the time of World War II. For example, penicillin, the first practical antibiotic, did not come into use until 1940. Given the dismal state of medicine until the mid-1900s, how did our ancestors manage to remain healthy for so many thousands of years? Did indigenous societies know something about mind and body, something very ancient that we had forgotten and were now trying to rediscover in the laboratory?

The concept of psychosomatic illness is now well established, but it originally was associated with hypochondria — "it's all in your head." The very real effects of the mind on the body have been confirmed by research. In a sense, we all became experts at developing psychosomatic disease very early in life. At the age of six I could create the symptoms of a cold in minutes if I did not want to go to school. Psychosomatic disease goes against every survival instinct programmed into the body by three hundred million years of evolution. How powerful the mind must be to override all of these survival and self-preservation mechanisms. Imagine if we could marshal these resources to create psychosomatic health!

In the last few decades the field of psychoneuroimmunology (PNI), which studies how our moods, thoughts, and emotions influence our health, has matured. PNI investigators discovered that the mind is not localized in the brain but rather is generalized throughout the body. Dr. Candace Pert found that neuropeptides, which are molecules that continually wash through our bloodstream, flooding the spaces in between each cell, respond almost instantaneously to every feeling and mood, effectively turning the entire body into vibrant, pulsing "mind." Our body as a whole experiences every emotion we have. The rift between mind and body had been resolved with the discovery of a single molecule. We also discovered how psychosomatic disease works. We know that when we become depressed every cell in our body feels it, our immune defenses are lowered, and we are more likely to become ill. We know that laughter, if not the best medicine, is near the top of the list. Years after I left the laboratory, PNI investigators discovered what shamans have long known, that the mind and the body are one. But investigators missed one element that is the crux of all shamanic healing: the Spirit.

THE QUEST FOR SPIRIT

By my mid-twenties I was the youngest clinical professor at San Francisco State University. I was directing my own laboratory, the Biological Self-Regulation Lab, investigating how energy medicine and visualization could change the chemistry of the brain. We were able to increase the production of endorphins, the natural brain chemicals responsible for reducing pain and for creating ecstatic states, by nearly 50 percent utilizing the techniques of energy healing. My students and I were making fascinating discoveries, yet I was growing increasingly disenchanted. We could influence brain chemistry but did not have the slightest clue how to help a person suffering from a life-threatening disease regain her health. We were like children who discovered that we could mix mud and water and turn it into clay. I wanted more than that. I wanted to discover how to build adobe houses, or at the very least to make pottery.

One day in the biology laboratory, I realized that my investigations had to get bigger instead of smaller. The microscope was the wrong instrument to answer the questions I was asking. I needed to find a system larger than the neural networks of the brain. Many others were already studying the hardware. I wanted to learn to program the system. If there were experts alive who knew how to draw upon the extraordinary capabilities of the human mind to heal the body, I wanted to find them. I needed to know what they knew. Anthropological stories hinted that there were peoples around the globe who claimed to know such things, including the Aborigines in Australia and the Inka in Peru.

A few weeks later I resigned my post at the university. My colleagues thought I was mad, that I was throwing away a promising career in academia. I traded my laboratory for a pair of hiking boots and a ticket to the Amazon. I set off to learn from researchers whose vision had not been confined to the lens of a microscope, from people whose body of knowledge encompassed more than the measurable, material world that I had been taught was the only reality. I wanted to meet the people who sensed the spaces between things and perceived the luminous strands that animate all life. I wanted to study with investigators who knew the energy side of Einstein's equation $E = MC^2$.

My research would eventually take me from the Amazon rain forest to the Andes Mountains in Peru, where I met Don Antonio, then in his late sixties. He was poor by Western standards. He had no television, not even electricity. But he claimed to have tasted infinity. "We are luminous beings on a journey to the stars," Don Antonio once said to me. "But you have to experience infinity to understand this." I remember smiling when the medicine man first told me how we were star travelers who have existed since the beginning of time. Quaint folklore, I thought, the ruminations of an old man hesitant to face the certainty of his death. I believed that Don Antonio's musings were akin to the archetypal structures of the psyche as described by Carl Jung. Antonio interpreted his myths literally, not symbolically, as I did. But I didn't challenge him then. I thought of trying to explain to my very Catholic grandmother that the Virgin Mary did not really have a virgin birth, that this was a metaphor for Christ's having been born enlightened, the Son of God in the fullest sense of the word. She would never accept it. For her the virgin birth was a historical fact. I believed the same to be the case with Don Antonio's musing about infinity. For both a nice metaphor had turned into dogma. The mythologist Joseph Campbell used to say that reality is made up of those myths that we can't quite see through. That's why it's so easy to be an anthropologist in another culture—everything is transparent to the outsider, like the emperor's new clothes.

At times I attempted to show Antonio that the emperor *was* naked, that he was confusing mythology for fact. That is, until I sat with him while he helped a missionary to die.

> *Tucked into a hillside, the village was built around and incorporated a substantial Inka ruin. Sections of the city's granite block walls were so expertly cut and fitted together that friction alone had held them in place for centuries.*
>
> *Near the edge of the altiplano the Inkas had built a hamlet, an outpost of their civilization. Now, a thousand years later, their descendants lived among ruins, farming the terraces that sloped down the hill from their village. In the courtyard, chickens, pigs, and a llama grazed. An Indian woman was grinding maize in one of the mortars. An old man led us to one of the huts. The shadows were growing long, and it took a moment for our eyes to adjust to the darkness of the room. A woman, her head covered by a black shawl, stood holding a candle and murmuring at the head of a bed, a pallet supported by two wooden crates in the center of the room.*
>
> *There was a woman lying there, stretched out on the pallet, an Indian blanket pulled up to her chin. It was impossible to judge her age, she was so emaciated. Her skin was yellow with jaundice and stretched taut over the bones of her face; the tendons in her neck were sharp ridges. Her hair was short and gray; her eyes stared blankly at the ceiling from hollowed-out sockets. She made no movement, no telltale sign of awareness, nothing to show us that she knew we were there.*

Antonio turned and looked at me, held up the candle, and I stepped forward and took it. He passed his hand over her face, and her eyes remained fixed on the ceiling. A silver crucifix at the end of a string of rosary beads lay on her chest and around her neck.

"A missionary," he whispered. "She was brought here two days ago by the Indians from below." He gestured toward the hillside and beyond it, toward the jungle.

"Her liver has failed," I said. "I think she is in a coma." I asked what we could do.

"Nothing. She will die tonight. We can only help to free her spirit."

Twenty or thirty candles had transformed the mud-and-straw hut into a sort of chapel. I sat on a sack of corn husks by the door and watched my companion, seated across the room from me. The room was warm from so many candles, insulated from the cool of the evening by its thick adobe walls.

He moved to the head of the bed and, ever so gently, lifted her head and removed the rosary beads from around her neck. He placed the beads in the palm of her left hand and closed her fingers around them. Antonio then signaled for me to blow out the candles.

I moved to the little ledge that ran like a shelf around the room while the old Indian chanted a low, murmured song. I looked back over my shoulder and his eyes were closed, his hand on her forehead, and his lips moved almost imperceptibly. There were three candles illuminating the room, and the smoke from those snuffed hung in the air.

Don Antonio moved his hands to a spot an inch or so above her heart. With first and second fingers extended, he began to make a counterclockwise circular motion, and he drew his hand away, still spiraling, up into the smoky air. Heart chakra. He did this three times, then started on the third chakra, beginning at a spot half an inch from the surface of her skin above her solar plexus, a perfect circle, three inches in diameter, slow, then faster, spinning up and away. He moved onto the deep hollow at the base of her throat, her stomach, her forehead, and then the top of her head.

"Look," he said.

I took my eyes from his face and looked down at the body, at the ever so slight rise and fall of her chest. Then Antonio hit me in the head.

It was lightning fast. His elbow came up and struck my forehead with a hard, sharp blow. My head swam for an instant. My hand flew to the spot reflexively.

"Look," he said.

It was an instant, nothing more. Something glimmered along the surface of her body, something milky and translucent an inch or so above the body's contour. Then it was gone. He took my arm with a firm hand and brought me around to the head of the bed.

"Look now. Soften your focus."

And there it was. Out of focus, but clearly there, an ever-so-subtle glow now three to four inches from her skin, as if a luminous mold of her body were emerging from the flesh. I had to concentrate not to focus. I felt an involuntary chill snake up my back.

"Am I really seeing this?" I whispered.

"Oh, you are seeing it, my friend," the old Indian replied. "A sight that we have forgotten, that has been clouded by time and reason."

"What is it?"

"It is she," he said. "It is her essence, her luminous body. She would call it the soul. She wants to let go."

Antonio worked on for another hour. He repeated the procedure that I had witnessed before, repeated it with the same patient intensity, never hesitating, dedicated to the work at hand.

Then he bent over her head, his lips less than an inch from her ear, whispering. Suddenly her chest heaved, and she gasped as the air rushed through her mouth and into her lungs. It stayed there.

"Exhale!"

And there came a long wheeze, like a labored sigh, as her last breath seeped from her chest, out through her open mouth. As though out of the corner of my eye, I suddenly saw the milky luminescence lift and coalesce into something amorphous, without specific shape, something translucent and milky like an opal hovered there over her chest. I saw the shape hovering over her throat, her head, and then it just wasn't there. A sense of great peace filled the hut.

"What was it?" My voice was a whisper.

"What the Inka call the wiracocha.*" He drew down her eyelids with his fingertips. "I'm glad you saw it."*

FROM VILLOLDO AND JENDRESEN,
Dance of the Four Winds.

Today, more than twenty years later, I have come to understand the old Indian and his claim that one can taste infinity. I've learned that the experience of infinity can heal and transform us, and that it can free us from the temporal chains that keep us fettered to illness, old age, and disease. Over the course of two decades with the shamans in the jungles and high mountains of the Andes, I would discover that I am more than flesh and bone, that I am fashioned of Spirit and light. This understanding reverberated through every cell in my body. I am convinced that it has changed the way I heal, the way I age, and the way I will die. The experience of infinity is at the core of the Illumination Process, the essential healing practice in this book.

HEALING VERSUS CURING

During my studies with the shamans I found that there is a difference between curing and healing. Curing is remedial and involves fixing whatever outer problem arises, such as patching a tire if you have a flat, or treating snakebite, or using chemotherapy to control a tumor. It does not help you avoid the nails on the road, the snakes in the woods, or the disease that caused the tumor. Healing is broader, more global, and complete. Healing transforms one's life, and often, though not always, produces a physical cure. I have seen many medical cures in which healing did not occur. I have also seen instances in which there was great healing but the patient passed away. Healing results from an experience of infinity. While healing, we measure success by increased well-being, by a sense of newfound peace, empowerment, and a feeling of communion with all life.

A few weeks after the incident with the missionary, while hiking in the mountains near Machu Picchu, I came down with a case of pneumonia. A full course of antibiotics did not help to control the infection, and the coughing fits simply would not stop. Every time I coughed, my abdominal muscles would go into spasm. I came to Don Antonio in acute pain. The old Indian asked me to lie down on a fur throw that he kept at the foot of his bed. He sat on a cushion by my head and performed a healing on me. He called on the four cardinal directions, then invoked Heaven and Earth. Next he raised his arms, as if he were parting the air above his head, and slowly brought them down by his side, as if he were expanding the edges of an invisible bubble. He repeated the motion, this time extending the edges of this invisible bubble forward to cover me like a blanket. I felt an immediate sense of safety and comfort. The chatter inside my mind ceased, and I slipped into a state of stillness and tranquillity I had felt before only during meditation. I could hear Antonio's voice from far away, instructing me to breathe in rhythm with him, and felt my breath accelerating to keep pace with his. I could feel his fingers turning in a counterclockwise direction around the hollow at the base of my throat, drawing out a sticky, cotton-candy-like substance. I noted all of this casually, as if it were happening to someone else, or as if I were seeing it in a dream, none of it disturbing my calm. And then my left arm began to twitch involuntarily. "That's the toxic energy leaving your system," Don Antonio said. "Don't be afraid. Let it happen naturally." The twitching then spread to my left shoulder and down to my right leg. It was completely involuntary, like the sudden jerking one sometimes experiences before falling asleep, except that this kept on going and building in intensity. Then, as suddenly as it had started, it stopped, and I fell asleep.

Nearly one hour had passed by the time I awoke and looked at my watch. Antonio was still sitting by me, his hands cradling my head. He asked me how I felt. I took stock of my body and realized I was unable to move. Strangely, though, the realization did not bother me. I felt as though I were floating in a warm, silent sea. Antonio began to massage my scalp, and after a few moments I was able to stretch my hands and feet and sit up. I felt as if I had had a solid night's sleep, and the pain in my chest was gone. I asked Antonio what he had done. "This is called *Hampe*, or energy healing," he explained. "You have spent most of the last hour in infinity," he added with a smile, "but that is only a figure of speech, for one cannot spend a measured amount of time in timelessness."

He treated me for only one session, yet almost immediately my cough subsided. My immune system had been kick-started, and I felt I was on my way to recovery. Even more important was a deeper healing that went far beyond my cure. After the healing session I was left with an abiding calm and serenity that I could only describe as a state of grace, of forgiveness and blessing, that has remained with me for years. I had tasted freedom from the chains that kept me bound to time past, to my painful history, to guilt, and to regret, as well as to my hopes and my anxiety about the future. I had tasted peace. I was brought up to believe that such grace was attained only through prayer and the generosity of God's love.

"I am not bestowing grace or any such thing on anyone," Don Antonio was quick to explain. "I merely held a sacred space in which you experienced infinity. You did the actual work yourself." He was letting me know that he had created the sacred space where healing happens. The energy within that space and the assistance from luminous beings in the Spirit world empowered me to heal myself.

The way of the shaman, I discovered, is a path of power, of direct engagement with the forces of Spirit. I had never experienced the path of power before. In my Christian upbringing I had learned to pray and would recite my evening prayers without fail. Later I studied meditation. Both prayer and meditation remain important practices in my life today. But the path of power is different. It requires a direct experience of Spirit in its own domain, in infinity. Tremendous healing takes place when we commune with the powerful energies of the luminous world. In the process, you shed your identity with your limited self and experience a limitless oneness with the Creator and the Creation.

The healing practices I learned and refined with my Indian mentor are ancient technologies that create sacred spaces where miracles can happen. They allow one to step into infinity and experience illumination in the timeless moment. This is the core shamanic healing practice in this book, the Illumination Process. When we enter infinity, the past and future are stripped away and only the here and now exists. We are no longer bound to the painful stories from our past, and our future is no longer scripted by our history. It is not that the past is magically wiped clean. The loss, pain, and sorrow we have lived through remain only as a memory; they no longer define who we are. We realize that we are not our stories. And the experience of infinity shatters the illusion of death, disease, and old age. This is not a psychological or spiritual process only; every cell in our body is informed and renewed by it. Our immune system is unbridled, and physical and emotional healing happen at an accelerated rate. Miracles become ordinary, and spontaneous remissions, those mysterious and baffling cures that confound medicine, become commonplace. And a spiritual liberation or illumination takes place. In the presence of infinity we are able to experience what we were before we were born and who we will be after we die.

The shaman with whom I studied believed that he could track his luminous nature — what we call the soul — through time the same way that he could track a deer through the forest. He claimed to have followed the luminous threads of his being as far back as the Big Bang at the beginning of time, and into the future, tasting who he was becoming, and beyond, to when our universe will again return to that singularity from which it was created.

The experience of infinity should not be confused with eternity. Eternity means an endless number of days. Eternity is bound to time, to growing old and dying. Infinity is prior to time itself and existed before time was born. And since infinity was never born, it is undying. Our infinite self is prior to life and death and never enters the stream of time itself. It was not born with your body, and it will not die when your body perishes. In infinity you exit linear time and move into the sacred. Because you no longer identify yourself within time exclusively, and with a physical form that ages and perishes, death no longer threatens the end of your days. This state of liberation is at the heart of many of the world's mystical traditions. Shamans discovered practical methodologies to achieve this goal. My mentor understood that his luminous nature was enduring. We want to believe and even suspect this to be true, yet very few of us know it with such certainty. Reading about it in a book does not count. Antonio once explained to me that for the shaman there is a difference between acquiring information and having real knowledge. Information is understanding that water is composed of two atoms of hydrogen and one atom of oxygen, H_2O. Knowledge is comprehending the nature of water so well that you can make it rain.

Over the years Don Antonio and I would develop and refine the Illumination Process, founded on a healing practice that was nearly destroyed by the conquistadors and the Church. The Illumination Process allows us to taste infinity and renew ourselves from the source that animates and informs all life. Of course, if you scrape your shin, you don't need to have a spiritual epiphany; you simply clean the cut and put a Band-Aid on it. But if your immune system is not responding, or if a loved one is faced with a life-threatening illness, or if you are repeating the same painful life patterns over and over, perhaps it is time to look beyond the concrete, beyond the finite, and into a healing practice founded on the experience of infinity.

CHAPTER 2

THE LUMINOUS HEALERS

During lunch Professor Lancho told us the history of the giant markings on the desert floor. As chief archeologist of the Nazca region, he is the most powerful man in the area. He approves every archeological dig, and has a police unit under his command to ensure that the sites aren't looted. I've known him for years. When he arrests temple looters he confiscates their booty, which goes to the regional museum. The grave robbers go to jail. Some of the pieces they unearth are thousands of years old. When he comes across an artifact that he thinks I will like, he saves it for me. It works like that in Latin America. He doesn't represent the law. He is the law. And we are friends. Today he gave me a gift in a shoe box. "Not even the museums have something like this," he told me. When I opened the box I found the forearm of a mummy. Its wrist was tattooed with the markings of a high shaman-priestess. Lancho has given me some interesting artifacts in the past, but this one took the prize for the oddest. Antonio was not happy at the desecration of this shaman's grave. Tonight we are doing ceremony at the figure of a gigantic hummingbird etched on the desert. I'll bring it with me and bury it, return it to the Earth where it belongs.

We finished the ceremony at midnight. We had walked to the giant markings on the desert floor to receive the energy of hummingbird, which embodies the qualities that shamans must have for their epic journey. I placed the mummified forearm at the edge of the altar, a simple woven cloth containing Antonio's medicine stones. When we looked at it in the darkness, its fingers seemed to be moving, calling to us. Antonio closed his eyes and began singing and shaking his rattle. He turned to me. His kindly, deep-set brown eyes had become transfigured, and I thought I was looking into the eyes of a hawk. "She is suffering," he said in a resolute voice. "She is tormented for her people, who were massacred by the Spanish many years ago at this place. We must help her." And he opened the ceremony again and began whistling and singing for their spirits to come.

Antonio couldn't believe his eyes. A string of entities appeared before us, scores of spirits lining up in the desert in front of the altar. Antonio ministered to them, telling each that it was time to rest, to return to their home in the Spirit world. He called on the lineage of medicine men and women — luminous spirits — to come and assist them, and one by one they were released from their pain. "She cannot be in peace until she knows her people have been mourned and healed," he said. As each spirit approached I thought I could sense its pain: a child who lost his mother and father, a young woman who lost her beloved, a man who lost his home.

This went on all night. At daybreak, as the last of the spirits was healed, Antonio instructed me to bury the forearm. "Now she can find her peace," he said. "That's why she was given to you by the archeologist. She arranged this all from the other side. She knew we would be here today and help her people heal."

The workings of spirit are sure strange...

JOURNALS

I WAS THE FIRST NORTH AMERICAN ANTHROPOLOGIST TO HAVE EXTENSIVE contact with the Q'ero nation, the last remaining Inka, who live in isolated mountaintops in the Andes. They still speak the pure Q'echua language, and have had little contact with either the church or the state in the last five hundred years. Their shamanic practices have remained intact since the time of the conquest, undiluted by the teachings of the missionaries. The Q'ero are the legendary keepers of the Inka prophecies. Their medicine people, including my mentor Don Antonio, believe their spiritual lineage extends back a hundred thousand years, and they remember stories handed down from grandmother to granddaughter that tell about the days before the coming of humans. The spiritual wisdom of their ancestors included lessons about life, the journey beyond death into infinity, and techniques for healing through the Luminous Energy Field.

The wholesale destruction of the Indians by the early settlers of the Americas obliterated the spiritual traditions of most native groups. The healing practices that survived the Indian genocide were carefully guarded. Understandably, the Native American shamans grew reluctant to share their heritage with the white people. The Spanish conquistadors, and the missionaries who accompanied them, destroyed the healing schools in Cusco. The temples were demolished, and churches were built on the same grounds using the original temple stones. The Inka healing traditions were no longer maintained by an organized order of shaman-priests, who were assiduously persecuted by the Inquisition. The Inka spiritual and healing practices were transmitted orally. When the Catholic Church outlawed the rites and ceremonies of Pagan peoples, the spiritual teachings became like a tapestry buffeted by the winds of time. All that remained after five hundred years were fragments closely guarded by the remaining shaman-healers.

We imagine that the Inquisition is a thing of the past, that this brutal organization ended with the arrival of the Age of Enlightenment, and this is largely true. The Inquisition shut down its offices many years ago except in one country, Peru, the land of the Inka. To this day, the last remaining office still operates under the direction of the Dominicans, the Catholic order that sentenced Joan of Arc to death. It is known as the Office for the Extirpation of Idolatries. It persists in the Andes because it is the only land in the Americas where the shamanic practices still thrive on a large scale. Today Peru is a Catholic country, with twenty-four million people. More than twenty million of these are Indios, who have been converted to Catholicism yet continue to seek healing from the shamans and greet Inti, the Sun, in much the same way as they did five hundred years ago.

That the Inquisition still maintained an active office in Peru was enough to draw my attention to the descendants of the builders of Machu Picchu. The idea that these medicine people still spoke with rivers and trees and conversed with God made them even more appealing. The possibility that shamans might have keys to ancient practices for healing mind and body made them irresistible. Thus began an endless journey that has taken me through the primeval garden of the Amazon rain forest to the highest peaks of the Andes. There I discovered an ancient spiritual practice that stated that each one of us was capable of experiencing infinity, and that this experience could make us whole; that the Earth does not belong to us but rather that we belong to the Earth; and that we can still speak with God and hear God's voice in all of Creation.

Under Don Antonio's guidance, I went back to the roots of the Inka civilization itself to collect the vestiges of a five-thousand-year-old energy medicine that heals through Spirit and light. Scattered throughout the remnants of the empire were a number of sages who remembered the ancient ways. Don Antonio and I traveled through countless villages and hamlets and met with scores of medicine men and women. We distilled the essence of their rituals. The lack of a written body of knowledge meant that every village had brought its own flavor and style to the healing practices that still survived. We traveled to the Amazon, and for more than ten years I trained with the jungle medicine people. We trekked the coast of Peru, from Nazca, site of gigantic markings on the desert floor that depict power animals and geometric figures, to the fabled Shimbe lagoons in the north, home to the country's most renowned sorcerers. In Lake Titicaca, the Sea on Top of the World, we collected the stories and healing practices of the peoples from which, the legends say, the Inka were born. When my mentor became too old to travel, I continued the search.

Antonio and I reconstructed the many threads of the Inka healing traditions. He compared it to reweaving an ancient tapestry that had been frayed by time and the European conquest. This was a tapestry that the conquistadors believed they had shredded beyond repair and scattered to the four corners of the crumbling Inka Empire. After nearly twenty-five years of research, we had only to knot these threads onto the loom of the living shamanic knowledge and reweave the parts of the fabric that had been torn by time. What emerged was a set of sacred technologies that transform the body, heal the soul, and can change the way we live and the way we die. They explain that we are surrounded by a Luminous Energy Field whose source is located in infinity, a matrix that maintains the health and vibrancy of the physical body.

Among the sages we worked with were Doña Laura, a highlands medicine woman, and Don Manuel Quispe, the eldest of the Q'ero medicine men. Each of these sages represented one of the roots of the Inka people, whose ancestors came from the coast, the jungle, and the highlands. Many of these masters have since passed away, but Don Manuel, at the age of ninety, remains my teacher today. As an anthropologist, I believe it's important to make one's sources verifiable and transparent. This has been my objection to authors whose work lacks credibility, since no one except they have met their sources. In the following pages I want to introduce you to the medicine people who guided my training. Each of these individuals is a self-realized shaman. Their work has become the stuff of legends. They were my teachers.

DON ANTONIO MORALES

Antonio was on the staff at the university in Cusco. I was looking for a translator to assist me in my field study, someone who spoke Q'echua, the Inka language, fluently and would be able to understand and translate the subtle nuances employed by the shamans. Professor Morales fit the bill perfectly. A thin, slightly built man who wore secondhand suits tailored in the 1940s and carried a plastic pen protector on his shirt pocket, not only was he fluent in Q'echua, he was a scholar able to decipher the poetry and philosophy of the Indio. But he had an innate dislike of anthropologists, whom he considered modern-day conquistadors come to plunder the spiritual bounty of his people. I had no idea at first why he agreed to work with me. He refused to take any money for his translation services, accepting only his room and board when we traveled. It was not until years later that I understood. I was to become his interpreter. He saw me as a bridge to bring the teachings of the shamans to the Western world.

It wasn't until the incident with the missionary that I discovered that Don Antonio led a double life: university professor to the *civilizados*, shaman-healer to the Indians. He wielded a rattle and feather as dexterously as a pen. Respected as a scholar, feared and loved as a shaman, he was the healer I was searching for, and he had found me. Antonio had been orphaned at an early age and had been raised by nuns. He grew up cleaning the churches of Cusco during the day and teaching himself to read and write at night. During the winter, which is the dry season in the Andes, he would depart to the mountain village of Paucartambo, to the Q'ero highlands, where he would continue his studies in the medicine way.

There are numerous ways that a shaman is called to his or her path. The most direct and deadly is lightning. Antonio had been struck by lightning at the age of twelve. Part of his right earlobe was gone, and a scar ran across his chest from his right shoulder to his left hip. For nearly two years after this incident he did not talk, and the nuns became convinced that he was feeble-minded. Yet by the age of fifteen he had read all the Western classics and was fluent in Latin and Spanish. The lightning bolt had rewired his brain and awakened dormant abilities that allowed him to fit perfectly among the university-educated mestizos in Cusco and the full-blooded mountain Indios. I'm convinced that the lightning strike left his brain extremely finely tuned, like a high-performance automobile that could run only on high-octane fuel. This meant he could not tolerate alcohol, and he would become tipsy after half a beer. His tongue would loosen, and he would begin to tell me stories of his youth. It was only during these times that he would answer all of my questions. The problem was that by the time he finished his first beer he would stop speaking altogether and fall asleep.

Antonio was the most unusual person I have ever met. I had not seen him for several years when I returned to Cusco with a group of my students. He had heard I was in town, and set out walking from his village at three in the morning to come to see me. Even at the age of seventy he refused to take buses and had the strength and agility of a cat. He arrived at the rustic posada we were staying in shortly after six in the morning. He entered the room without knocking, trying to surprise me. I looked from the shower and saw him leap like a cat into the air and land on my still-sleeping roommate, Hans, a friend and Chinese martial arts master. I closed my eyes, dreading what would happen to my old teacher. When I opened my eyes I saw the two of them standing on the bed, shaking hands and laughing like old friends.

Antonio was a seventh-level *kurak akuyek*, the highest degree that a shaman can attain.* He had taken me on as an apprentice, yet considered me an equal in the ways of the West. He was convinced that shamanism no longer belonged to the Indio, that the West needed the sacred teachings to forge a new philosophy and ecology into the twenty-first century. He hoped that I would prove him right.

---

* The first level of Andean shamanism is the *ayni karpay*, where the student comes into proper relationship with nature and is not yet considered a shaman. The second level is the *pampa-mesayok*. *Pampa* refers to the lowlands; the *mesa* is the shaman's altar; and *yok* means power. At this level, the apprentice becomes a *mesa* carrier. She has assembled her collection of medicine objects, and her duty is the stewardship of the Earth. The third level is the *alto-mesayok*, or high *mesa* carrier. The responsibility of the *altomesayok* is to the *apus*, the sacred mountains, and the medicine teachings. There are three degrees within this level, and as your power and wisdom increase, you come under the protection of progressively higher

DON MANUEL QUISPE

Don Manuel Quispe is ninety years old and the oldest living Inka medicine man. I first read about Don Manuel in a 1962 *National Geographic* special on Peru, where he was described, at the age of fifty-two, as one of the oldest of the Q'ero shamans, and the only one who still remembered how to count with the *quipu*, the ring of colored knotted strings on which the accounting of the Inka Empire was kept. By the time I met him in 1989 all that he could use the *quipu* for was telling stories. He had forgotten the math of the Inkas. All that remained in his head were the legends.

Don Manuel was born in the community of Q'ero, the son of a farmer. At the age of fifteen he became very ill. His father took him to the healers of his village, and no one was able to help, not even the doctors at the medical post in the city of Cusco. While bringing his emaciated son back to Q'ero, he stopped at the sanctuary of Huanca, a holy place where the power of nature congregates. The sanctuary of Huanca was so revered by the Inka that the Catholic priests had built a church above it to convert the Indians. A miracle occurred, and Don Manuel began to eat and regain his strength. Huanca is located halfway up the southern face of Mt. Pachatusan, whose name means "axis of the world." The mountain spirits instructed Manuel to travel to another *apu*, or sacred mountain, named Ururu, directly across the valley. Young Manuel spent the next few months living in a cave like a hermit, drinking the water that filtered through the walls of the cavern, going for long walks alone in the mountains. Here is where he

---

mountains. The fourth level is the *kurak akuyek*. The word *kurak* means "elder," and *akuyek* means "to chew" or "to masticate." Like a mother who chews a grape before feeding it to her child, at this level the shaman "chews" the knowledge so that others can "digest" it. It can take a lifetime to reach this level, where your duty is to the stars. Few shamans attain it. The levels above it are known as the *Inka Mailku*, or ancient of days; the *Sapha Inka*, or resplendent one; and *Taitanchis Ranti*, or one who shines with the God-light within. Each of these levels is more refined than the ones below and is recognized by the powers that the shaman acquires.

first began speaking to the *apu*. The mountain itself became his teacher. He had been on the brink of death, had experienced the continuity of life on the other side, and come back. On his return to Q'ero he completed his apprenticeship, formally undergoing the rites of passage under one of the legendary shamans of Q'ero.

When I first met him he had already lost all of his front teeth. He knew my mentor Antonio and agreed to teach me. All he wanted from me was a new set of teeth. The ordeal was more complicated than I ever thought possible. The dentist had to extract the remaining teeth a few at a time, and he would be in pain for days after each surgery. Twice he nearly died under the anesthetic. And he held me responsible for each painful extraction. Finally he got his new dentures, looked at himself in the mirror, and smiled. The next week he began to teach me everything he knew. We went to Mt. Ausangate and he gave me his *hatun karpay*, or great transmission. And then he told me to go jump into Otorongo Warmi Cocha, the female-jaguar lagoon.

I looked at him, incredulous. "Do what?" I said.

"Go jump into the lagoon," he replied. "That's for all the pain from having my teeth taken out."

We were at fourteen thousand feet, it was the middle of winter, and a light snow was falling around us. The thermometer on my backpack read ten degrees below zero. The water in the lagoon came from a blue-ice glacier in the middle of the pool. At that temperature and altitude, I was convinced, I would have a heart attack.

"It's not my fault that your dentist didn't give you enough anesthetic," I said, trying to persuade him to find another test for me.

"I nearly died at the foot of the mountain before the *apu* gave me back my life," he said, a thin smile revealing his shiny new teeth. "I've brought you to the holy mountain. I'm giving you my *karpay*. Let's see if the *apu* gives you your life." And then he explained that I would have to touch my lips to the ice at the bottom of the pool. Although the blue ice was only six or seven feet under the water, I doubted I could hold my breath long enough to touch bottom.

"Don't stay in long," he said.

I'm too old for this, I thought. But something inside me had taken over, and I found myself stripping down: mountain jacket, fleece pants, thermal underwear. The cold was biting through my skin. I hovered on a boulder above the icy water, clasping my arms tightly over my chest, my skin all goose bumps. Thinking about it wasn't helping. I dove into the pool and had the breath knocked out of me by the frigid water. I managed to swim to the center of the pool but couldn't hold my breath long enough to dive. Then I went under, as if in a dream, and kissed the glacier.

Afterward Don Manuel explained to me the initiations of the Andean shaman. There are seven levels or major rites of initiation. The healer needed only the first two levels; the master shaman needed the first four. Very few people completed all seven levels. Don Manuel, Doña Laura, and Don Antonio were the only remaining shamans who had achieved all seven levels of initiation.

In the first level the medicine person receives the seven archetypes or organizing principles of the universe, embodying the spirits of serpent, jaguar, hummingbird, and condor in their four lower chakras. In the upper chakras the student receives three luminous beings, the organizing principles of the lower, middle, and upper worlds. They also obtain the "bands of power," a protection for the healer, so that they will not pick up any toxic energies from their clients. They then undergo the *kawak* rite, which opens their eyes to the shaman's way of seeing. I've adapted this rite into a technique (see Chapter 5) to awaken the Second Attention that allows one to perceive the luminous side of life.

The second level in the Andes is the *pampamesayok*. During this rite the shaman receives a lineage of medicine men and women dedicated to the stewardship of the Earth and all sentient beings. After this rite of passage the healer never works alone. She is supported by a community of luminous spirits who assist her in healing. These luminous ones transcend culture and time. The rite connects you to this lineage of luminous healers who recognize you and respond to your call.

"There was really no need to go into the lagoon," Don Manuel said as I sat shivering, trying to put my clothing back on. "I was only testing your determination."

That night, while Don Manuel slept, I stole into his tent and hid his teeth. It took him two days to find them.

For nearly seven years, until he became too frail to travel, Don Manuel and I taught the ways of the *kurak akuyek* to my students in North America. The high point of our travels came when we performed a ceremony for healing the Earth at the main altar at the Cathedral of St. John the Divine in New York, the largest Gothic cathedral in the world. Hundreds of people attended. Don Manuel grinned the entire evening. He had never imagined he would be holding ceremony at a Christian altar.

DOÑA LAURA

Doña Laura was Antonio's medicine partner. They had learned their art in the highlands from the same teachers. He had moved to the city. She had moved even farther into the mountains and lived above the snow line near Mt. Ausangate, the Inka holy mountain. She was a fierce old crone, one of the most frightening people I have ever met. She could look right through you, and by candlelight her features seemed to transform, her nose becoming a hooked beak, her eyes turning into those of a falcon. She disapproved of Antonio's teaching me, and she scolded him that these were the ways of the Indio. It was only after I had completed my rites of passage, after I became a *kurak akuyek* myself, that she stopped calling me "boy" and we became friends.

I never took her contemptuousness personally. She was fierce with her own students, beating them with a stick when they committed particularly stupid mistakes. And getting a smile from her, however brief, was worth more than praise from any other teacher. She was the head of the medicine societies, of equal rank and stature as Don Antonio. And she was a shape-shifter. Whereas most shamans could travel in the shape of a spirit eagle or jaguar in dreams, Laura could do it while awake, in broad daylight. She could merge with a condor and fly the giant bird according to her will, diving into ravines or flying miles above the ground, contemplating the landscape below. Once, at the base of Mt. Ausangate, she was challenged by one of her students, a short, pudgy Indian fellow named Mariano who had a great sense of humor and a knack for gathering medicinal plants but who managed to do most everything else wrong. "How do I know you are really inside the body of the condor and not imagining it?" he asked. I was a dozen feet away, at our camp with Don Antonio. The air suddenly became electric, and I saw a faint smile cross Antonio's face. We all knew better than to challenge the old woman, and all of us were waiting intently for her response.

"Is there a difference between reality and imagination?" she answered in a gentle tone. We looked disappointedly at each other.

It was getting close to dusk, and a half dozen of us set out to collect brush and *masto*, the dried llama droppings that are used for fuel so high in the mountains. Half an hour later we were all back at camp except Mariano. Most of Laura's students were women, and they had given the two male apprentices women's names, which they used when they were not around. "Where is María?" they taunted playfully. "Maybe she has gotten lost," one snickered.

I could tell that Antonio was getting worried. It was wintertime on the second highest mountain in South America. In a half hour the temperature would fall below freezing. He motioned to me and another man to go search for him. As we were setting out we noticed Mariano staggering toward camp. His face was bloodied, and he was barely able to stand. I carried a first-aid kit, which I kept stowed at the bottom of my bag, for situations like these. My mentor did not like to use Western medicines, but at that altitude no medicinal plants grew.

We were so far above the tree line that no plants of any kind were to be seen. We were surrounded by a barren, icy landscape punctuated by patches of bare rock. We brought Mariano into our tent and saw that the back of his jacket had been slashed; the white filler was stained red with blood. The gash had gone through his clothing and torn his skin, leaving three deep gouges on his back, like those made by the talons of an animal. We asked Mariano to tell us what happened, but all he would do was shake his head and say that he had fallen and cut his face on the ice. Later that night we overheard him apologizing to Doña Laura. It seemed that a giant condor had swooped down from the sky and tried to carry him away. Condors have been know to abduct a fully grown sheep, fly several hundred feet into the air with the animal in their clutches, and drop it to its death on the rocks.

Over the years Doña Laura and I became friends. One day she told me that the secret of shape-shifting was to realize that you were no different from anything else in the universe, no better and no worse. Once you understood in your cells that you were exactly the same as everything else, no more important than an insect, no less important than the Sun, you could change into any shape you wanted, whether a condor or a tree. You could even become invisible to others. She explained that the shaman had to master the art of invisibility in order not to call attention to herself. Antonio had mastered this. He was invisible to the Catholic Church. No one knew who he was, so he was free to change the world. "You can accomplish anything," she once told me, "as long as you are willing to let others take credit for it."

DON EDUARDO

Eduardo Calderón was a fisherman. He lived in the North Coast region of Peru, near the fabled Shimbe lagoons, and had a natural gift for seeing the luminous nature of life. Eduardo was the descendant of Moche Indians, a great civilization that thrived a millennium ago. He developed his gift through years of training, and he could look at you and recite the story of your life, both the public story that you wore on the surface as well as the more intimate, secret stories that each of us carries. Don Eduardo's reputation as a seer and healer has spread throughout Peru. Even members of the Senate had come to see him.

Antonio had indicated on a number of occasions that I should travel to work with Don Eduardo. The coastal shamans were renowned for their ability to see into the Spirit world. This was an art that had been lost in the Andes. Most relied, rather unskillfully, on reading coca leaves. I did not respond very enthusiastically to Antonio's suggestion. I had my hands full training with him, and I already was spending time in the Amazon learning the Death Rites and the journey beyond death. And then Antonio disappeared.

I had flown back to Peru to spend three months traveling the highlands with him. He had taken a sabbatical from the university, and no one knew where he had gone or when he would come back. It was the rainy season in the Amazon, which made traveling there impossible. Reluctantly I packed my bags and went to visit Don Eduardo, whom I had worked with several years earlier. The day after I arrived he was scheduled to perform a healing ceremony. There were twenty-five or thirty people, the sick and their families, gathered in a circle at night on the beach. Eduardo had an assistant on either side. After about an hour I felt a need to stretch my legs, so I walked down the beach. When I returned to the circle, I noticed that one of Don Eduardo's assistants was gone. The man had become ill and lay wrapped in a blanket. Eduardo motioned for me to come to his side and take the assistant's place.

As soon as I sat next to Don Eduardo I felt I had entered another more lucid and crystalline world. It was as if someone had turned on the lights and I could see. The luminous shapes that I had seen in the Andes with Don Antonio paled in comparison. When I walked a few feet away, the world became filled with the darkness of night once again. Don Eduardo's Luminous Energy Field was making my seeing crystal clear. He then turned to me and told me that I had a gift, but that I had to train it, to learn to see with clarity and precision.

That night, for the first time, I saw an intrusive entity. This spirit was lodged inside a woman's Luminous Energy Field. The parasitic entity was sucking her life force. She had come to Eduardo complaining she was depressed and in despair. The healer stood up, took a sword and crystal from his altar, and proceeded to extract the intrusive entity that was causing this woman's ailment.

"We have to heal it," he said as he turned toward me. "This is her brother, who was killed in an automobile accident a few months ago. He doesn't know that he is dead, and he has come to his sister for assistance."

He then performed a healing for the deceased brother, to help him awaken from the nightmare he was in and complete his journey to the Spirit world.

"A priest would have done an exorcism and tossed this soul back into the dark," Don Eduardo said.

That night my eyes were opened to a world I had previously refused to accept. I had believed naively that only angels and luminous beings inhabited the Spirit world. The last thing I wanted to discover was that physical and emotional conditions can be caused by invasive spirit entities. I wanted nothing to do with the "lowlifes" of the Spirit world. But I did want to learn to see. And Don Eduardo was a master seer. What I saw taught me that a person does not automatically become holy because he has died. There are as many troubled people on the other side as there are in the physical world. Eduardo taught me the rites of passage that awaken one's ability to see into the invisible world. This was a piece of the puzzle that Antonio and I had long been searching for, the *kawak*, or "seer," rites.

CHAPTER 3

THE LUMINOUS ENERGY FIELD

I've found that the San Pedro potion does nothing other than make me sick. The slimy liquid reminds me of mucus, and I choke when I try to swallow it. Must be an acquired taste...I've run the numbers, and there is not enough active ingredient in the potion to make me or anyone in the ceremony see visions. I'm convinced that the altered state I'm in is created by Don Eduardo's singing. And then there is the energy that he claims enters the ceremonial space when he summons the spirits of serpent, jaguar, hummingbird, and condor. I'm not convinced that it's not all a subtle form of hypnosis, that he is taking us on this joyride, and that his clients get well because they want to and receive the shaman's permission. Posthypnotic suggestion. I once saw a man strip down to his shorts in front of a full auditorium because of a posthypnotic suggestion.

What I can't explain is the fact that I'm seeing energy. It only happens when I sit next to Don Eduardo. When I go more than a few feet away from him I sense nothing. It's like he is surrounded by an electric space, where the air actually tingles. When I'm inside his space I see everything he sees.

Last night he was treating a young woman. She was standing six feet in front of us, holding her child, and Eduardo began to sing. Suddenly there were five or six tendrils, like the arms of an octopus, coming out of the woman's belly. One of these arms reached out and connected to the belly of a milky form we saw by her side. Eduardo described this entity as her former husband, who was trying to take custody of her daughter.

"This man is hurting you," Eduardo said. "He is joined to you through your womb."

Although a hefty man, the shaman sprang from behind his medicine stones, took hold of one of the swords in his altar, and landed next to the woman. When he touched the tip of the sword to the woman's abdomen, her entire luminous body lit up. It was the eeriest sight, like a lava lamp that had suddenly been turned on, and the globs swirled in currents of light and dark, streaming a few inches above the surface of her skin. Then, with a flick of the sword, he severed the dark cord, which retracted immediately into the entity's abdomen. Right into its gut.

Eduardo began sucking the other dark tendrils from the woman's belly, loudly drawing into his mouth the toxic strands. He did this for nearly a minute and then stepped outside the circle. I could hear him retching violently.

When I looked at the woman again, all of the dark fibers were gone. I could see her second chakra spinning sluggishly and then picking up speed, reorganizing itself into a conical shape. Then Don Eduardo returned to the altar and plopped down next to me, exhausted.

"Did you see, compadre?" he asked.

JOURNALS

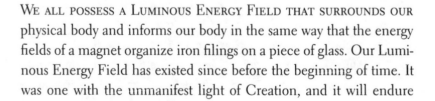

WE ALL POSSESS A LUMINOUS ENERGY FIELD THAT SURROUNDS OUR physical body and informs our body in the same way that the energy fields of a magnet organize iron filings on a piece of glass. Our Luminous Energy Field has existed since before the beginning of time. It was one with the unmanifest light of Creation, and it will endure throughout infinity. It dwells outside of time but manifests in time by creating new physical bodies lifetime after lifetime.

Imagine you are enveloped in a translucent, multicolored orb pulsing with blues, greens, magentas, and yellows, enfolding you to the width of your outstretched arms. Just above your skin, streams of golden light shimmer and flow through the acupuncture meridians. Between your skin and the membrane of the Luminous Energy Field swirl resplendent currents that fuse into whirlpools of light. This reservoir of vital force is a sea of living energy as indispensable to our health as the oxygen and nutrients carried by the bloodstream. They are the energies of the Luminous Energy Field, the purest and most precious fuel for life. When the vital reserves in the Luminous Energy Field are depleted through illness, environmental pollutants, or stress, we suffer disease. We can ensure our health and vitality and extend our active, healthy years by replenishing this essential fuel.

Indian and Tibetan mystics who documented the existence of the Luminous Energy Field thousands of years ago described it as an aura or halo around the physical body. At first it seemed odd to find the same concept of a human energy field among the jungle and mountain shamans in the Americas. Once I grasped the universality of the human energy field, however, I understood that every culture must have discovered it. In the East, mandalas depict the Buddha enveloped by blue and gold bands of fire. In the West, Christ and the apostles are shown with luminous halos around them. In the mystical literature, the Apostle Thomas is said to have glowed with the same radiance as Christ. Native American legends speak of persons who shimmered in the night as if lit by an inner fire. The Andean storytellers recall the ruler Pachacutek, considered to be a Child of the Sun, who sparkled with the light of the dawn.

Every living thing on Earth is composed of light. Plants absorb light directly from the sun and turn it into life, and animals eat green plants that feed on light, so that light is the fundamental building block of life. We are light bound into living matter. Every living thing around us is made of light, bound and packaged in different forms and vibrations. Physicists studying subatomic particles know that when you look deeply enough into the heart of matter, you find the entire universe is made up of vibration and light.

We are mistaken if we believe that the accounts of the light around the Buddha or Christ are merely myths and legends. Nor can we attribute these individuals' radiance to some strange bioluminescence produced by the body, as if it were a kind of firefly effect. The Buddha showed us the way to enlightenment. He taught us to follow our light to attain liberation from suffering. A blinding radiance was said to appear over Christ as he was baptized in the Jordan River. When we believe that Christ may have glowed with the light of His love but that *we* certainly cannot, we negate Christ's teachings when He said, "Even greater things than I have done, you shall do." We commonly consider these references to the light as metaphors. We seek illumination as some form of higher understanding. My investigations have convinced me that the ancient references to the light are facts that can be verified through experience. Then, when we understand our luminous nature, we can shun the trappings of the material world and experience infinity. First, though, we need to understand the anatomy of the Luminous Energy Field.

THE ANATOMY OF THE SOUL

The Luminous Energy Field is an invisible matrix that informs the anatomy of the body. When I was in grade school I felt awed by the beautiful oval patterns created in iron filings on a sheet of glass by the invisible fields of a magnet. I noticed how, when I moved the magnet under the glass, the iron filings dutifully followed like a caravan of metallic ants. Moving the iron filings with my finger, I saw that when I let go they rushed back immediately to their original positions. It almost seemed as if the filings had a mind of their own. What caused the little bits of iron to return to their original pattern? Many years later I understood that Western medicine, in an effort to change the physical body, was merely moving the iron filings around the glass. Surgery and medication often brought about violent, traumatic change on the body. This approach struck me as crude and invasive, like scattering the iron filings with my hand, rather than moving them by shifting the magnet underneath the glass.

The magnet with the iron filings above it became a metaphor for me of how matter and consciousness are linked through an invisible energy field. I have seen how after a surgeon excised a tumor the cancer returned weeks or months later. While the physical mass, the tumor, had been removed, the Luminous Energy Field still contained the blueprint of the illness. It was only a matter of time before the disease recurred, rushing to reestablish itself according to the preexisting pattern. When we heal through the Illumination Process we change the iron filings of the body by changing the energy fields that organize them. We heal the Luminous Energy Field, and the physical body follows.

The Luminous Energy Field has four layers extending outward from the body. They are:

1. Causal (the Spirit)
2. Psychic (also known as etheric—the soul)
3. Mental-emotional (the mind)
4. Physical (the body)

Each layer stores a different quality of energy. The outermost layer stocks the energy that fuels the physical body. The layer beneath stores the energies that sustain our mental and emotional stamina. Underneath this layer are the refined psychic energies, and closest to the skin is the finest energy of all, our spiritual fuel reserves. The mystical literature refers to these layers as "subtle bodies." In reality, they are not separate from each other, in the same way that the colors of the rainbow are not disconnected but rather dissolve into one another.

The Luminous Energy Field contains an archive of all of our personal and ancestral memories, of all early-life trauma, and even of painful wounds from former lifetimes. These records or imprints are stored in full color and intensity of emotion. Imprints are like dormant computer programs that when activated compel us toward behaviors, relationships, accidents, and illnesses that parody the initial wounding. Our personal history indeed repeats itself. Imprints of physical trauma are stored in the outermost layer of the Luminous Energy Field. Emotional imprints are stored in the second layer, soul imprints in the third, and spiritual imprints in the fourth and deepest layer. Imprints in the Luminous Energy Field predispose us to follow certain pathways in life. They orchestrate the incidents, experiences, and people we attract to ourselves. Imprints propel us to re-create painful dramas and heartbreaking encounters, yet ultimately guide us toward situations wherein we can heal our ancient soul wounds.

I am not too concerned with the layer in which an imprint is located, in the same way that I'm not very concerned where a letter is stored in my computer's memory. I'm interested in editing and changing the content of the letter. In a similar manner, during the Illumination Process I'm interested in clearing the negative content of an imprint. All imprints contain information, which inform the chakras, which then organize our physical and emotional world. The information in an imprint organizes the Luminous Energy Field, which later organizes matter.

The Luminous Energy Field contains a template of how we live, how we age, how we heal, and how we might die. When there is no imprint for disease in the Luminous Energy Field, recovery from an illness happens at tremendous speed. By the same token, imprints for diseases can depress the immune system, and it can take an extremely long time for us to regain our health during an illness. None of us wants to spend months convalescing when we could have recovered in a matter of days or weeks. When we erase the negative imprint that caused the onset of illness, the immune system can rapidly eradicate the disease.

George, an athletic man in his early twenties, suffered from a malfunctioning kidney. Once a donor had been located, George came to

LAYERS OF THE LUMINOUS ENERGY FIELD

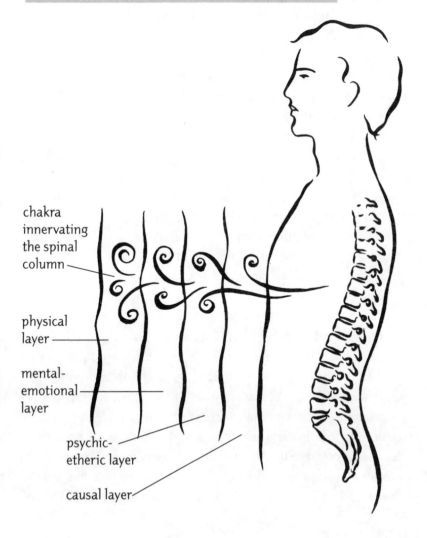

chakra innervating the spinal column

physical layer

mental-emotional layer

psychic-etheric layer

causal layer

the University of California Medical Center in San Francisco for a transplant. The day before his operation he was given drugs to suppress his immune system, so that his body would not reject the foreign kidney. As a standard precaution before any transplant, the organ was carefully examined to make sure no cancer cells were piggybacking along. A few cancer cells did slip by, and within a week these had grown into tumors the size of grapefruits. George looked grotesque and was in a great deal of pain.

His doctors took him off the immune-suppressing drugs. White blood cells rushed to the area, and within days the tumors were eradicated. The problem was that his immune system was rejecting the kidney. The immune suppressants were resumed and the kidney began to take, but again the grapefruit-size tumors returned. This went on for several weeks, during which time the tumors flared up seven times. After two months of on-again-off-again treatment, his body finally accepted the kidney well enough that George could go off the medication, and the cancer was eradicated. I believe that George recovered so quickly because he did not have the blueprint for cancer in his Luminous Energy Field. His immune system speedily eliminated the tumors once he was taken off the immune-suppressing drugs. The cancer never returned.

RIVERS OF LIGHT

The Luminous Energy Field is shaped like a doughnut (known in geometry as a torus) with a narrow axis or tunnel, less than a molecule thick, in the center. In the Inka language it is known as the *popo*, or luminous bubble. Persons who have had near-death experiences report traveling through this tunnel in their return voyage to the light. The human energy field is a mirror of the Earth's magnetic field, which streams out of the North Pole and circumnavigates the planet to reenter again through the South Pole. Similarly, the flux lines or *cekes* of the Luminous Energy Field travel out the top of the head and stream around the luminous body, forming a great oval the width of our outstretched arms. Our energy fields penetrate the Earth about twelve inches, then reenter the body through the feet.

Although the strength of the Earth's magnetic field drops off very rapidly the farther it travels from the planet, it never actually reaches zero. It extends for hundreds of miles into space before diminishing in strength, and travels at the speed of light, at about 186,000 miles per second, to the edge of the Universe. The human energy field appears to extend only a few feet beyond the body since, like the magnetic field of the Earth, it diminishes in strength very rapidly. Yet it also travels at the speed of light, connecting us to the luminous matrix of the entire Universe, known to the Inka as the *texemuyo* or all-pervading web.

Along the surface of the planet run flux lines or *cekes*, similar to the acupuncture meridians, connecting the major chakras of the Earth. The meridians of the Earth traverse the globe, transporting energy and information from one part of the planet to another. Shamans claim they can communicate with each other through the luminous matrix formed by the flux lines of the Earth. The medicine person is able to sense and sometimes see the luminous grid of the Universe extending beyond the Earth into the galaxies themselves.

Many people in our technological society are disconnected from the matrix of the Universe. I often find that people who come to see me with the symptoms of chronic fatigue have become totally disassociated from the natural world. They do not go for walks in the woods, plant tomatoes in their gardens, or even stop to smell the flowers. This is not to say that walking in the forest will cure chronic fatigue syndrome, which is a complex medical condition. Yet people who suffer from this condition require vital reconnection to the natural grid as part of their healing.

As the flux lines run along the body of the Earth, the acupuncture meridians run along the surface of the skin, connecting acupuncture points (which are in essence very small chakras) to each other. These energy meridians are analogous to the circulatory system inside the body. They are the veins and arteries of the Luminous Energy Field. Medicine people of the Americas know the meridians as *ríos de luz*, rivers of light that flow within the luminous body. Legends say that five thousand years ago the first practitioners of acupuncture were able to see the meridians webbing the surface of the body. Even today, most of the renowned acupuncturists in Japan are blind. Their acclaimed diagnostic skills are possible because they are not distracted by physical appearances. Able to follow the flow of *chi* with their fingers, they sense its rhythm and pulse along the acupuncture meridians. By sensing where the *chi* is blocked and where it is flowing vigorously, they are able to diagnose health or disease.

Mystical traditions abound with references to individuals who can perceive the Luminous Energy Field. Among the Inka they are known as the *kawak*, the seers. In the Nazca plains in the southern desert of Peru there is an abandoned city known as Kawachi (the name means "place of the seers"), an entire town dedicated to training individuals to sense the luminous nature of life. Over the years I developed the ability to perceive the streams of light that flow through the luminous body, and read the imprints of health and disease. I believe that this is an innate ability that we all possess but either do not develop or lose after the age of seven or eight because we are taught to believe that the material world is the only "real" world. Shamans throughout the Americas rely on their ability to perceive the energetic realm.

Nearly twenty years ago, while visiting the city of Cusco, the capital of the Inka Empire, I had the opportunity to observe a healer named Maximo as he ministered to an Indian woman. The old woman suffered from asthma and was beset by coughing fits upon even the slightest exertion, such as climbing a flight of stairs. After the usual greetings and introductions, Maximo asked the woman to sit down and unbutton her blouse. He circled to her back, where he began to trace with his forefinger an invisible line on one side of her spine. He would stop, push the fingertip deep into her flesh, and instruct her to relax. The healer continued to trace lines down her back, applying pressure at various points as the woman flinched with pain.

Maximo had stimulated the exact points used by acupuncture for the treatment of asthma. After the therapy I expressed my amazement, and the healer's reply astonished me even more. He claimed that he had never heard of acupuncture or of any such points. He explained that he had learned this technique from his grandmother, who taught him to see the rivers of light or *cekes* along the surface of the skin, and to massage the points where it was blocked so that the light could flow freely again. As his last patient for the day was leaving, I asked Maximo if he could describe these rivers of light so I could better understand them. He smiled, asked me to strip down to my shorts, and with a bright red lipstick belonging to Anita, his wife, proceeded to draw the rivers of light on my body. I was standing on the dining-room table while Maximo took my photograph when Anita and their two daughters walked into the room, screamed, and ran out of the house. I would later find out she was not as shocked at the sight of a half-dressed man on her dining-room table as at the fact that we had used her only lipstick. On my return to California I compared the photographs with charts of the Chinese acupuncture meridians and found that they coincided exactly. For Maximo and other shamans in the Americas the rivers of light in the body are tributaries that flow into and draw their substance from the great luminous rivers that course along the surface of the Earth.

THE CHAKRAS

People are often surprised that the chakras exist in the Native American traditions. "I thought the chakras were Hindu," people often say to me. The chakras are part of the anatomy of the Luminous Energy Field. Simply because kidneys were named by Europeans does not make the kidney exclusively European. Similarly, the chakras are not exclusively Hindu.

Every living being has chakras. Crickets have them, as do deer, squirrels, and humans. Even trees have chakras. The chakras in animals run along their spine, as they do in humans. A tree's chakras, on the other hand, are mobile, as trees lack a spinal column. You can scan the surface of a tree with your hands. When you feel the tingling sensation that indicates the presence of a chakra, take hold of it with both hands (they are about the size of a basketball). By gently nudging its chakra to align with one of your own chakras, you can connect energetically with the tree.

In parts of South America the chakras are known as *ojos de luz*, or eyes of light. My Inka mentor called them *pukios*, or light wells. We receive impressions of the world through our chakras, perceiving love in our heart; sexuality, fear, and danger in our belly (second chakra); and insight in our brow chakra (sixth). In a disagreeable situation, our second chakra can go into spasm and we may feel a knot in our stomachs. From the unmistakable experience of sensing feelings through the heart center, we come to associate love with the heart, or refer to sadness as heartache.

In the Eastern traditions there is an assumption that the chakras are contained within the human body. For the shaman, however, the chakras extend luminous threads, or *huaskas*, that reach beyond the body, connecting us to the trees, the rivers, and the forests. These luminous fibers also extend to the places where we were born and live and to our personal history and our destiny. While the Hindu tradition describes seven chakras, the shaman that I trained with taught me to perceive two additional ones: the eighth chakra, above the luminous body but within the Luminous Energy Field, known as the *wiracocha*, or source of the sacred; and the ninth chakra, outside the body, at one with all of Creation and residing in infinity, in the world of Spirit, known as the *causay*, the point of the unmanifest Creation — infinity. We will explore the chakra system in greater detail in Chapter 6.

The chakras are the organs of the Luminous Energy Field. They are swirling disks with wide mouths that spin a few inches outside the body, through which they drink in the radiant fuel stored in the luminous body to nurture us spiritually, emotionally, and creatively. The narrow, funnel-shaped tip hooks directly into the spine. The chakras transmit information of past trauma and pain, contained in imprints in the Luminous Energy Field, into the nervous system. The chakras inform our neurophysiology, affecting our moods and influencing our emotional and physical well-being. The chakras also connect to endocrine glands that regulate all of human behavior.

LIVE LONG AND RADIANTLY

When the Luminous Energy Field becomes toxic as a result of environmental or emotional pollutants, the chakras become clogged. The process is analogous to an engine whose pistons are mired in sludge. The chakras build up residues and begin to spin sluggishly, so that we have no energy and become easily irritated or depressed. Eventually they seize up and our immune system breaks down. The quality of the fuel reserves in the Luminous Energy Field also influences our longevity. When our energy reserves become toxic, the chakras convey these toxins to the central nervous system, and we can succumb to disease or be in danger of dying. How effectively we renew our energy stores can determine how healthy and active we remain. The quality of our luminous energy stores can even influence how we age.

Scientists who study aging have discovered that the biological clocks in the body do not run on linear time. Our cells do not have a limited number of years; instead they have a limited number of lives, a limited number of times that they can replicate and make accurate copies of themselves. Say, for example, that liver cells can make a hundred copies before they begin to break down. If you were to freeze a handful of liver cells after forty-nine replications and thaw them out in the laboratory a hundred years later, they would still continue to divide another fifty-one times. While each liver cell may have one hundred lifetimes, your eating habits and lifestyle will greatly influence whether or not you get to enjoy the full length of this life span. If you consume excessive amounts of alcohol, you might reduce the life span of your liver. Equally as important to our longevity as lifestyle and diet is the quality of the reserves in the Luminous Energy Field. Although no laboratory evidence correlates the reserves of the luminous body to the lifetimes of cells, shamans believe that the quality and purity of these vital energies are a determinant of longevity. When we are under emotional or physical stress, we deplete these reserves very rapidly. Our fuel stores drop dangerously low. The Luminous Energy Field, like a battery, can operate at full tilt for only so long before it is unable to regenerate itself. We all know of people who aged very suddenly after a traumatic incident in their lives — say, after the breakup of a marriage or the loss of a loved one. How well we preserve and regenerate our luminous reservoir seems to govern how long and how healthily we will live.

One way to upgrade the reserves in our Luminous Energy Field is through the Illumination Process, described in Chapter 7. Another way is by cleansing our chakras. It is practiced in the morning while in the shower. Hold your left hand at the base of your spine, and with your right hand three or four inches above the skin feel for your first chakra. (See Chapter 4 for the location of the chakras.) Spin the chakra counterclockwise (imagine that your body is the face of the clock) three or four times, rotating your fingertips in a circle. Rinse your fingers in the water. This eliminates the sludge and toxins that adhere to the walls of the chakra. Repeat for all seven chakras, making sure to rinse your fingers thoroughly in between. Try to sense the dense energy — like cotton candy — on the chakras. Now go back to your first chakra, spinning it clockwise three or four times. Repeat for all seven chakras. This exercise increases the speed of the chakras, allowing each energy vortex to spin at its optimal frequency. A clean chakra is able to draw in natural energy to replenish the reserves in the Luminous Energy Field and keep us in exceptional health.

The Illumination Process can also be used for achieving super-longevity. Biologists sometimes compare the aging process of cells to the making of a photocopy of a photocopy of a photocopy. By the ninety-ninth copy, the image begins to grow fuzzy. Sometime in our late thirties our skin begins to lose its elasticity, the crow's feet around our eyes become more pronounced, and age lines begin to appear. If only we could find the original image and duplicate it! Through the Illumination Process we can copy from the first image; we can inform our bodies from that original source that informs all of life. The same source that informs the redwood trees and the spiral arms of the Milky Way is available to inform us when we practice healing through the Luminous Energy Field.

IMPRINTS OF HEALTH AND DISEASE

The Luminous Energy Field contains information that can kill us or heal us, in the same way that DNA encodes within its double helix the formulas for longevity as well as the inherited health conditions that plague us. It holds the blueprint of our body just as an architectural drawing holds the design of a house. But unlike a physical blueprint, which is separate and remains intact as the house ages, our luminous template is continually informed by both the positive and negative incidents we experience during our lives. Unresolved psychological and spiritual traumas become engraved like scratch marks in our luminous fields. Positive experiences do not leave a mark in our luminous body. The peace and serenity we discover through our spiritual practice is fuel for the innermost layers of the Luminous Energy Field, energizing the soul and the spirit.

The blueprint that shaped and molded us since we were inside our mother's womb contains the memories of all of our former lifetimes—the way we suffered, the way we loved, how we were ill, and the way we died. In the East these imprints are known as karma, forces that sweep through our life like a giant tide that we cannot swim free of. These imprints contain instructions that predispose us to repeating certain events from the past. We want to learn where these energy imprints are located in the Luminous Energy Field and how to erase them so that the body, mind, and spirit can return to health.

In the outermost layer of the Luminous Energy Field is the membrane or "skin" of the luminous body. This membrane serves as a defensive cocoon in the same way the skin is the protective membrane of the body. The imprints of physical trauma and disease are etched onto this membrane like designs cut into glass. When I work with a client suffering from a prolonged illness, I almost always find an energetic imprint depressing the immune system. If the imprint is not cleared, recovery can take months or years, and the person not only will be predisposed to a recurrence of the same condition but will carry the imprint into her next lifetime. Imprints etched into the emotional-mental layer of the Luminous Energy Field predispose us to live in particular ways and to become attracted to certain people and relationships. These imprints dictate the course of our emotional lives. It is very difficult to change our lifestyle without clearing the imprints in this layer. Imprints stored in the etheric or soul layer inform and organize our physical reality. Imprints in the causal or spiritual layer choreograph our journey through life, including the kind of spiritual peace and fulfillment that we will attain.

An imprint stored in the luminous body and a letter stored in a computer's memory bear similarities. You can take a screwdriver to your hard disk drive, yet no matter how closely you scrutinize it, you will not find any sentences, punctuation, or paragraphs. The language of computers consists of magnetically charged zeros and ones.

The Luminous Energy Field is similarly coded. Childhood abuse is not recorded as an image of a child being battered. Likewise, a cancer does not appear like a blob in the energy template. They both appear like pools of dark, stagnant energy to those who can see. When an imprint is activated, it launches its programs, fueling them from the energy stores in the Luminous Energy Field. It's nearly impossible to stop. It's like entering a river on a raft. Once you push off into the white water, there is no going back. You have to shoot through the rapids before you find another spot to come ashore.

Imprints are formed when the negative emotions that accompany trauma are not healed. One client had a highly charged imprint produced when her father and mother separated. Susan was seven at the time, and she believed that it was her fault that her father had left, that she must have done something wrong. She was struggling with severe abandonment issues, which did not surface until two years into her marriage, when the imprint was suddenly activated. Although she loved her husband and he had never given her cause to doubt him, she was convinced that she could not count on him, or any man, to be supportive when she really needed him. There was nothing her spouse could do to reassure her. When I scanned her Luminous Energy Field, I perceived a bundle of knotted strings, like a tangled ball of yarn, clustered above her left shoulder. When an imprint is active, it begins pulsing within the Luminous Energy Field. Susan's was vibrating above her shoulder. Years of psychotherapy had helped her to understand her issues of abandonment, but therapy could not clear the imprint. Crises or emotional stress would trigger the script contained within the imprint, which would begin to play itself out again. Her abandonment issues would surface and be projected onto every male in her life. After three sessions Susan was able to begin trusting her husband to be supportive of her. She has forgiven her father and repaired her relationship with him.

However, I have seen clients who have suffered physical and emotional abuse, including victims of rape and wartime torture, who did not develop imprints in their Luminous Energy Field. They were able to heal the pain and negative emotions that accompanied the trauma. We all know people who have suffered tremendous loss, accepted the challenges and lessons of life, and grown from them. We also know persons who have been permanently scarred by pain and trauma. They remain deeply wounded, bitter, and resentful. How is it that the psychiatrist Jerome Frank was able to find meaning and purpose while interned in a concentration camp during World War II, after his family had been killed by the Nazis? If we are able to heal the emotional component of a painful situation as it is happening, an imprint is not created in the Luminous Energy Field. When we discover compassion and forgiveness in the midst of our pain, no residual toxic energies are absorbed into the Luminous Energy Field.

Imprints in the Luminous Energy Field can arrange strange and apparently unrelated events in the outside world. They can orchestrate our meeting love partners who all have the same toxic personality traits. They can strand us in the oddest places to come upon someone we are destined to meet; they can program us to be in the vehicle hit by oncoming traffic or in the one that just missed the accident. The story of Magda illustrates how imprints in the etheric or soul layer of the Luminous Energy Field can organize the physical world as readily as they can create disease within the body.

Magda came to see me suffering from what she described as "terrible bad luck." She was a single mother when her only son, then seventeen years old, had been involved in a tragic automobile accident. Every year on the date of his death Magda would find herself in a life-threatening situation. One year her car was rear-ended while she was stopped at a traffic signal, and she had to be taken in for emergency surgery. The following year a case of indigestion sent her to the emergency room, where she was given an oral solution of barium for an exam. The doctors discovered that she was allergic to barium only when her heart stopped. This pattern continued for five consecutive years. Magda could not understand why she kept experiencing near-death trauma that occurred only on February 26.

When Magda first walked into my office she exclaimed, "Why couldn't it have been me who died? Why do I have to continue to live?" She blamed herself for allowing her son to go driving with his friends that evening. Without him she felt alone, with no purpose in life or any reason to continue living. During the Illumination Process Magda experienced muscle twitching, cramping, and physical release in her body. Several times she wept softly while her body shook. Toward the end of one of our sessions she reported a deep sense of calm, claiming that she felt that her son was at peace, that she had felt him next to her, trying to comfort her. After a series of sessions, we cleared the imprints that predisposed her to these accidents, known in psychiatry as the anniversary effect. She had the realization that their souls were united. She was certain that she would never be separated from her son. Magda was then able to grieve the passing of her child and no longer continued to reenact his accident. She spent the next February 26 in fine health. When the energetic pattern was broken, the world around her changed.

When an imprint is activated, its toxic energy spills into a chakra, wreaking emotional havoc or compromising our immune response. In Magda's case, her suffering grew like dark storm clouds, which broke at the anniversary of her son's death. When I observe an imprint in the Luminous Body I first notice the storm clouds orbiting around it. These dark energies always indicate the presence of an active imprint. When it begins to play itself out, we gravitate to people and situations that will allow us to relive the circumstances of the original wounding in an attempt to heal it.

GENERATIONAL IMPRINTS

In the Amazon rain forest the medicine people speak about curses that befall families and that are transmitted from one generation to the next. In my years of studying with shamans I discovered that these healers were speaking metaphorically, referring to imprints that are transmitted between generations. The most common form of generational imprints are the physical conditions that we inherit from our mothers and fathers. We know that heart disease and breast cancer run in families. If your mother and grandmother died of heart disease, you have genetic risk factors that predispose you to heart ailments. These hereditary conditions are also archived in the Luminous Energy Field.

Ken originally came to see me about a marital problem. He and his bride were having difficulties adjusting to their new life together and wanted counseling. During our interview I noticed a dark spot in Ken's energy field, six inches above the chest. I scanned more closely and sensed what seemed like a root extending from this dark pool into Ken's heart. I asked him if there was a history of heart disease in his family. He replied that all of his relatives had good hearts and no one had died of heart disease. And he claimed to feel strong and fit. I was surprised, as I have learned to trust my seeing. I encouraged Ken to get a medical checkup and specifically a heart workup, to eliminate red meat from his diet, to exercise, and to take care of his heart. I went ahead and worked on his heart chakra, my rational mind telling me that perhaps he was suffering from emotional stress that I was misreading as a physical heart condition.

Three days later Ken called to say that his brother had just undergone an emergency quadruple heart bypass operation. During a routine physical exam doctors found his brother's heart on the verge of collapse. Ken's own medical checkup showed his heart was fine. Yet I knew that the Luminous Energy Field can reveal conditions months and years before they manifest in the physical body. I encouraged Ken to continue taking preventive measures to strengthen his heart. I also made sure that he received an Illumination in order to clear the condition at the source, before it manifested physically. Ken

healed himself before he needed to be attended to with heart bypass surgery.

SEVEN GENERATIONS

Imprints can also be associated with the psychological characteristics that we inherit from our parents. In Nancy Friday's book *My Mother, Myself*, she discovers she is reliving her mother's life despite doing everything in her power to do exactly the opposite. We often end up fighting the same battles and following the same life paths that our mothers and fathers did. If your grandmother and your mother were involved with abusive men in their lives, you might be predisposed to the same sort of relationship. Even the Bible states that the sins of the father will be inherited for seven generations. These sins are not judgments against innocent descendants but are negative energies that are passed along from one generation to the next. Psychologists believe that the subconscious motifs and behaviors we inherit from our parents might be encoded into the circuitry of the brain, and that the only way we can reprogram these circuits is through psychotherapy. I'm convinced that these negative patterns and habits are encoded in the Luminous Energy Field as well and that the Illumination Process can accomplish in one session what can often take years to heal through psychotherapy.

Talk psychotherapy often is not enough to achieve healing. Psychology believes that once you become cognizant of hitherto unconscious "complexes" and "drives," you can become free of their noxious influence. Shamans, on the other hand, believe that intellectual cognizance barely scratches the surface and is not enough to bring about healing. Knowing that she was sexually abused as a child will help a woman to understand her reluctance to trust men, but this understanding alone will seldom allow her to participate in an intimate relationship. We all understand that we should exercise more, eat fewer desserts, and meditate more often, yet we often have to compel ourselves to do the things that we know are good for us. The rational mind has very little influence over the emotions and our physical longings, fears, and desires. Breakthroughs can occur with the Illumination Process because this work operates at the causal level of the Luminous Energy Field. Talk therapy works only at the mental level and is unable to erase or reinform archaic imprints in the Luminous Energy Field.

There is another form of imprint that is handed down from one generation to the next, from father to son and from mother to daughter. I became curious about this when I saw it operating within my own family. My grandfather lost everything during the Great Depression at the age of forty-five. When my father was forty-six, a prosperous attorney in Havana, he lost his job and all of his worldly possessions when the Communists took over. My father had always measured his success by his material achievement—the kind of house he lived in, how much he earned, where his children went to school. When we fled Cuba after the revolution he determined to rebuild and again attain the level of material comfort he had once enjoyed. For the next twenty-five years he worked day and night, hardly seeing his family, depriving himself of the pleasures of life. Finally, in his early seventies, he retired to a life of relative comfort. A few months after his retirement he called and told me he had woken up that morning and did not know where his life had gone. That day he determined to begin living his life, and soon he embarked on a travel odyssey that took him to Europe, China, and other places he had always wanted to see. Still, though, he had lost a quarter of a century.

When my brother turned forty-eight, doctors discovered a very malignant type of cancer in his brain. Despite radiation and chemotherapy, he died a few months after his diagnosis, at the prime of his life, leaving two beautiful children and a wife. At the age of forty-five I also faced the loss of everything I loved. My earlier books had placed me in high demand as a speaker and teacher. Four days out of every week I was on the road lecturing on energy medicine and shamanism. I had very little time left for my family. Despite valiant attempts to preserve my marriage, including therapy and counseling, it fell apart. My wife and I separated, and shortly thereafter my six-year-old girl was thrown from a horse and had to undergo emergency surgery to repair a ruptured liver. I was leading an expedition to the Amazon jungle when this happened, visiting with a renowned medicine man — Don Ignacio. The shaman was a great seer, and when I explained to him what had happened in the last six months of my life, he described a dark mass over my heart.

"It's the grief that I'm feeling," I told him.

"No," he said as he gently placed his hand over my heart. "It is your grandfather's misfortune." He then went on to describe how my father's father had destroyed another man's career and incurred his wrath. This "curse" had been transmitted to my father, to my brother, and then on to me.

"You can heal this by battling adversaries in the world the rest of your life," Don Ignacio explained, "or you can heal your heart and the outer world will follow."

That evening Don Ignacio helped me to heal my heart. He cleared the dark nebula over my heart chakra and the generational imprint etched in my Luminous Energy Field. I flew back to the United States the following morning. My daughter was released from the pediatric intensive care unit a few days later and has recovered completely. It was too late to save my marriage, but my relationship with my children has grown and thrived. Today we have a great friendship. They have taught me how to be a great father. Since then I've become aware of how an imprint can be passed down from one generation to the next. When we heal these imprints within us, we heal them for our parents and children as well. I believe I've spared my son the need to go into major life crisis at the age of forty-six to heal his male lineage going back several generations. How do I know for sure? I know that I survived with my family intact, even though my marriage ended. Unlike my father, it did not take me twenty years to recover.

REIMPRINTING

For us believing physicists, the distinction between past, present, and future is only a stubbornly persistent illusion.

ALBERT EINSTEIN

The shaman is interested in draining the toxic emotional energy around an imprint and then erasing the imprint itself. The early stages of the shaman's training consists of a deep clearing or "scouring" of her Luminous Energy Field. The shaman no longer identifies with her personal history. Thus the Navajo medicine woman is able to say, "The mountains am I, the rivers am I." Shamans may have suffered loss, hunger, pain, and abuse, but they understand that above all they are travelers on a great journey through infinity.

This is the goal of healing through the Illumination Process. I am not very interested in working within my client's stories, the way the psychotherapist is. I am interested in assisting clients to realize that they are not their stories, not actors in a script written by their mother or father or by the culture or time they happen to be living in, but storytellers. To do this I have to access the underlying imprint in the Luminous Energy Field. It is very difficult to access these imprints directly. It's like trying to watch a movie by pulling the videotape out of its housing. We can only get to the film through the interface, in this case the VCR and the television screen.

The interface between our material world and the Luminous Energy Field is the chakras. In a sense, these spinning vortexes of

and physical aging is accelerated. When a shaman completes her healing process her chakras become clear. They spin freely and vibrate with their original purity again.

The Amazon shamans believe that when you clear all your chakras you acquire a "rainbow body." Each center vibrates at its natural frequency, and you radiate the seven colors of the rainbow. According to legend, when you acquire the rainbow body you can make the journey beyond death to the Spirit world. You are able to assist others in their healing, and you can die consciously since you already know the way back home. The jungle shamans believe death is a great predator that stalks each and every one of us. They say that many illnesses are caused by the death that festers within us. These medicine people believe that death (or lifelessness, as I prefer to think of it) claims us little by little, until one day we realize that we are more dead than alive. I've seen it happen to many persons, and I believe this condition is rampant in America today. When your chakras are clear you are no longer stalked by death. You are claimed by life, and therefore you can never be claimed again by death. The flag of the Inka nation is the rainbow, which holds a very special place in their mythology. You can see it flying over the rooftops of Cusco even today.

While the practitioners of yoga recognize seven chakras, Don Antonio taught me that we have nine chakras. Seven of them are within the physical body, while two are outside the body. He called the eighth chakra the *wiracocha*, which is the name of the Creator or Great Spirit (the word means "sacred source"). The eighth chakra resides within the Luminous Energy Field. It hovers above the head like a spinning sun. It is our connection with the Great Spirit, the place where God dwells within us. The *civilizados* (the whites as well as the Indios who have been exposed to Western beliefs) possess a dull, sooty sun for an eighth chakra. "It is because the *civilizados* have been kicked out of the Garden," one of their medicine women told me. Curiously, the Spanish word *Indios* means "one with God." For Indios who have not subscribed to Western mythology, the eighth chakra shines like a golden disk. We see this chakra illustrated as the light surrounding Christ and as the fire that descended upon the apostles at Pentecost, when they received the gift of the Holy Spirit. When we die, the eighth chakra expands into a luminous globe and envelops the other seven chakras in a vessel of light. After a period of atonement and purification, the eighth chakra manufactures another body, as it has done again and again over so many lifetimes. It leads us to our biological parents, and to the best life (not the easiest!) to acquire the experience we need to grow spiritually. The charged, traumatic memories of our previous incarnation are transfused into our next body as imprints in our Luminous Energy Field.

The eighth chakra's source is the ninth chakra, Spirit. The ninth chakra resides outside the Luminous Energy Field and extends throughout the cosmos. It is the heart of the universe, at one with the Great Spirit. My mentor believed that the eighth chakra was where God dwelled within us, and the ninth chakra that part of us that dwells within the Creator.

The eighth chakra corresponds to the Christian concept of the soul, which is personal and finite. The ninth chakra corresponds to Spirit, which is impersonal and infinite. The soul has always been the preoccupation of religion, which is concerned with its salvation. Because the soul is personal, it seems to be autonomous. We presume that we can either be at one with spirit or disconnected from it. The ninth chakra is one with all of Creation, infinite and eternal, in contrast to the finite, personal soul. I will refer to this center as the eighth chakra, given that the word *soul* has so many different connotations for us, from a kind of music to a type of food to a much-debated element of the self. The eighth chakra manifests in time. The Egyptians called it the *Ka*. The ninth chakra is present in the timeless now, a point without time, unfettered to history. It is immanent and transcendent, never dying and never having been born. The Egyptians referred to it as the *Khu*.

The chakras metabolize life energies from nature. All of our energy comes from five sources: (1) plants and animals, (2) water, (3) air, (4) sunlight, and (5) biomagnetic energy (known as *chi* in the East and *causay* to the Inka). These nutrients go from the most material food, such as animals and plants, to the most ephemeral, pure light and energy. We absorb plant and animal foods and water through the digestive tract, oxygen through the lungs, sunlight through the skin, and *causay* through the chakras. The luminous energies circulate through the chakras just as water and food, the physical energies, course through our bodies. When our digestive track is clogged, we cannot absorb the nutrients in foods. Similarly, when our chakras are blocked, we cannot ingest the *causay* stored in the Luminous Energy Field.

The chakras extend luminous threads that reach beyond the body, connecting us with trees, rivers, forests, and other people. Our chakras are coupled to our bodies for only a short while. At death they withdraw from the physical body and rejoin the eighth chakra, and our journey continues in the invisible world.

EARTH CHAKRAS

The five lower chakras, from the root to the throat, are nourished primarily by the Earth. Imagine a tree whose roots go deep into the ground. The nutrients it draws from the Earth are carried up the trunk to the highest branches. The sunlight it absorbs through the leaves is turned into energy that in turn is transferred all the way to the roots. The four upper chakras are fed primarily by the energies of the Sun, our star. The sky-god religions emphasize the development of the upper chakras to the neglect of the lower. The sky-god civilizations perfected technology, reason, and logic. The Earth-goddess religions emphasize the lower chakras to the neglect of the upper ones. These civilizations remained agrarian cultures with little interest in Western-style progress while achieving advancement in astronomy, philosophy, and architecture (the Chinese discovered gunpowder but used it only for fireworks; it took the Europeans to use it for warfare). I believe that today we must develop the gifts of both the Earth chakras and the sky chakras.

Like the organs in the body, each chakra performs a unique function. The first and second chakras digest emotional energies, churning them over to draw out nutrients. They can metabolize the energies from physical and emotional trauma and turn them into sources of power and light. Just as the digestive system draws out nutrients from food and returns the undigested roughage to the Earth, the lower chakras return to the Earth the heavy energies that they cannot metabolize into fuel. When the first chakra is disconnected from the Earth, the lower centers are unable to expel emotional wastes. There is no exit channel. These wastes turn into toxic sludge that adhere to the walls of a chakra and slow its spinning. When sludge builds in our second chakra (where the fight-or-flight response resides) we interpret the world as hostile and aggressive. The solar plexus, heart, and throat chakras (third, fourth, and fifth) are nurtured by the finer energies of love, compassion, and empathy. They are not equipped to digest emotions of any kind. (We get in trouble when we try to digest heavy emotions and feelings with our heart chakra — we get emotional heartburn.) The sky chakras are fed by the subtlest spiritual energy.

During my own training as a shaman I received a rite known as the "bands of power" in which my mentor wove invisible bands around my body. I make sure my students in the Healing the Light Body School receive the same rite, as it provides a very important spiritual protection for the healer. Five bands are installed at various levels of the body. The first band is black, representing the rich, dark Earth, and is woven over the first chakra. The second band is red, representing water, the blood of the Earth, and is woven over the second and third chakras. The next band is golden, representing fire, and is woven over the heart. The fourth band is silver, representing wind, and is woven over the throat. The final band is of pure white light, representing the *causay*, and is woven over the third-eye chakra. The bands are a link to the five elements and nourish the chakras with Earth, air, fire, water, and *causay* directly.

THE FIRST CHAKRA

ELEMENT: Earth

COLOR: Red

BODY ASPECTS: Physical foundation; elimination of wastes; rectum, legs, feet; testosterone and estrogen

INSTINCT: Survival, procreation

PSYCHOLOGICAL ASPECTS: Feeding, shelter, safety, ability to provide for oneself

GLANDS: Ovaries and testes

SEEDS: Kundalini, abundance

NEGATIVE EXPRESSION: Hoarding, predatory behavior, mindless violence, chronic fatigue, birth trauma, abandonment issues

The first chakra is located at the base of the spine, between the anus and the genitals. It is the gateway to the feminine, extending luminous filaments down our legs into the biosphere. Like a taproot reaching into the moist, rich places in Mother Earth, the first chakra supplies us with essential nutrients. It grounds us and is the foundation on which our luminous energy system rests. When we become disconnected from the Earth, we begin to get our life nourishment from the surface. As a result, we become like a tree whose shallow, widespread roots cannot keep it from toppling during a storm. We lose our stability, our foundation, and our security.

When the first chakra is disconnected from the feminine Earth, we can feel orphaned and motherless. The masculine principle predominates, and we look for security from material things. Individuality prevails over relationship, and selfish drives triumph over family, social, and global responsibility. The more separated we become from the Earth, the more hostile we become to the feminine. We disown our passion, our creativity, and our sexuality. Eventually the Earth itself becomes a baneful place. I remember being told by a medicine woman in the Amazon, "Do you know why they are really cutting down the rain forest? Because it is wet and dark and tangled and feminine."

First-chakra drives are primary and instinctual. We seek shelter. We forage for food. We strive to survive even under the most adverse situations. We procreate. These urges are fundamental instincts. In the same way that we can hold our breath but we cannot command our body to stop breathing, we cannot override our instinct to survive.

The four instinctual drives—fear, feeding, fighting, and sex—are mirrored in the agendas of the lower two chakras. These are the basic programs required for physical and emotional survival. The compulsion to overeat or to hoard money or toys is one of the negative expressions of the feeding instinct. We can never get enough to satisfy us. An unbalanced first chakra manifests in feelings of scarcity and lack. Even those who have a great deal may fear loss of their possessions. Ironically, the poor often are more generous than the rich. With a clear first chakra, the mentality of scarcity disappears. We come to realize that nothing is lacking and that we live in abundance. Intellectual understanding is not enough. We must know with every cell in our body that we are being cared for and sustained by the Universe. A collapsed first chakra makes us build fences to protect what we own from our neighbors. An unhealthy second chakra makes us gather piles of stones to defend ourselves from them.

Testosterone and estrogen are the hormones associated with the first chakra. Laboratory studies show that testosterone elicits two primary responses in the human male: sex and aggression. When women are given testosterone injections they complain that they cannot stop thinking about sex. An imbalance in the first chakra can exacerbate the effects of testosterone, causing a man to confuse the two instinctual impulses of this hormone. When that happens he begins to hurt the woman he loves and eventually destroys the intimacy in his love relationship. It leads to sexual abuse, which is widespread throughout not only America but also the rest of the world, particularly in countries making the transition from a village-based society to a city-based one. In South Africa, which is undergoing such a transition, a woman is raped every twenty-six seconds. When I work with a woman who has experienced sexual abuse early in life, I often find her first chakra shut down, many times from a subconscious fear that she might harm others as she was harmed by her father or another male in her family.

Estrogen, which is produced by the ovaries, is essential for maintaining bone mineral content. Estrogen production drops off dramatically after menopause, which can make a woman susceptible to osteoporosis. In nonindustrial societies women do not seem to have the high incidence of osteoporosis that we find in America. Some investigators argue that this is because women in the third world do not live as long and therefore never get to suffer significant bone mineral loss. I am convinced that another reason is that women in nonindustrial societies maintain an active connection with the feminine Earth throughout their lives. The first chakra induces in women powerful feelings of nurturing, desire for relationship, and mating. Imbalances in this chakra can result in a woman's overwhelming concern for security in her relationship at the cost of her autonomy.

Tribal cultures perform first-chakra rites of passage to celebrate a youth's coming into manhood or womanhood. The ceremony encourages the youth to release the parental bonds holding him to his mother and father. During the ceremony the youth claims the Earth as the mother who will never leave him and the Heavens as the steadfast, reliable, enduring father. This ensures that the young person will continue to be parented, but now by powers greater than his biological mother and father. The youth is now able to participate in ceremonies and offerings to Heaven and Earth, therefore maintaining a conscious connection to these cosmic parents. Lacking these rites of passage into puberty, Westerners are spiritual orphans. We struggle through life feeling motherless and fatherless, and later find that we do not know how to be dependable parents.

An individual operating out of the first chakra is in a state of primary fusion with the world. He is absorbed by the senses and engages the material world exclusively. He believes that the world owes him something and that those around him should recognize that he is special. He becomes self-centered and narcissistic. He cannot experience authentic love because he cannot put himself in the place of another; he is unable to "walk a mile in another person's moccasins." This center corresponds to the first seven years of life. The traumas experienced in these early years, including birth and prenatal trauma, are recorded in this chakra, forming psychological complexes that stunt later development. Like a young child, a person motivated primarily by the first chakra will be preoccupied with his needs for survival and entertainment. When cornered, he can become violent, lashing out physically or emotionally at the perceived threat. The first-chakra person will look for temporary sensual gratification at whatever cost. Often he cannot tell where his body ends and the world begins, so others become an extension of himself and cease to matter in his eyes. When I see a client who has suffered early childhood abuse or who was abandoned by one or both parents, I immediately look for first-chakra involvement. Former-life traumas are often located in the first or second chakra. Throughout history dictators seeking domination have been propelled by the negative drives of the first chakra.

There are remarkable positive attributes of the first chakra. Its survival instincts ensure the continuation of the species: They drive us to mate and bear children, and allow humans to persevere under the most adverse of conditions. In Sanskrit the first chakra is called *muladhara*, meaning "foundation." Our energetic house must be built on a strong footing. In yoga this chakra is thought of as the home of Kundalini energy. Its symbol is a coiled serpent asleep at the base of the spine. Kundalini is seen as the active power of the great goddess Shakti, the force that animates all creation. For the shaman this is the primordial serpent who swallows its own tail, Ouroboros, and portrays an unconscious state of self-absorption. To the Amazon peoples this power is represented by the *sachamama*, the water boa. In North America it is illustrated by the rattlesnake. As we clear the imprints within the first chakra, the Kundalini energy is awakened. The primal serpent uncoils, and its feminine energy moves up through the chakras. Shamans in the Americas, India, and Tibet have long believed that it is through the power of the primal feminine that all creatures move, live, procreate, and flourish. It's no surprise that the serpent was the one to bring us the fruit of the tree of knowledge in Genesis. Its energy, which lies dormant within each of us, is the energy of the Earth and the heartbeat of the mother planet.

THE SECOND CHAKRA

ELEMENT: Water

COLOR: Orange

BODY ASPECTS: Digestion, intestines, kidneys, urinary tract, sexual potency, adrenaline, lower back pain, menstrual pain, loss of appetite

INSTINCT: Sexuality

PSYCHOLOGICAL ASPECTS: Power, money, sex, control, fear, fighting, passion, self-esteem, sexual or emotional abuse, inherited parental issues, incest

GLANDS: Adrenals

SEEDS: Creativity, compassion, family

NEGATIVE EXPRESSION: Fear, fighting

The second chakra is located four fingers below the belly button. It is linked to the kidneys and to the element water. The second chakra activates the adrenals, the stress glands in the body. The adrenal cortex, or outer part of the gland, manufactures more than a hundred different steroids, including sex hormones. The medulla, or inner section, produces adrenaline, which tells the liver to release blood sugar, making us alert. Adrenaline is the hormone that mediates the fight-or-flight response. I mentioned earlier that the first chakra builds fences for protection, while the second chakra stockpiles rocks to defend itself. The problem is that we always need more powerful rocks to do the job. The other side always seems to have a bigger pile than we do, and the perceived threat escalates. The Cold War was a perfect example of second-chakra thinking on a global scale. When the United States entered into the Cold War, many were convinced that the Russians had bigger navies and better warplanes than we did. In reality the Russian navy was rusting and sinking, and its warplanes were no match for ours. The second chakra is the motivator of bullies and cowards. Bravado and posturing are inspired by this chakra. Imagine, if you will, the alpha-male display of the silverback gorilla baring his teeth and pounding his chest.

The second chakra metabolizes energy nutrients in the Luminous Energy Field. All forms of energy represent food to this chakra. It processes the Earth energy taken in through the first chakra and digests emotional energies in the nervous system. When this chakra is functioning properly, it can shred negative emotions such as anger and fear and expel them through the first chakra as waste. When this chakra is out of balance, these negative emotions fester within us, sitting in our gut, decomposing slowly. We all know people who are unable to let go of anger and carry resentment for weeks and even years. These negative emotions settle in the second chakra, turning it toxic. Eventually these emotional toxins are assimilated through the Luminous Energy Field.

The second chakra is home to passion. It expresses itself through creativity and intimacy. In the first chakra we reproduce. In the second chakra we make love to our beloved. The Sanskrit name for this center is *svadhisthana,* which means "dwelling place of the self." Chronologically, this chakra corresponds to the ages between eight and fourteen. Adolescent longing for romantic adventure originates with the surge of activity in the second chakra. This chakra is erotic, full of lust and fantasy, propelling high-adrenaline romance. If the adolescent does not develop a clear and positive sense of self during puberty, the growth of the second chakra can become stunted. This person will not develop robust emotional boundaries and will be unable to recognize that what others want may differ from what she desires. She may feel tormented by relationships and by people who can never meet her needs.

The negative expressions of the second chakra are anger and fear. Shamans believe that fear is the great enemy. It is a cunning adversary that you must not engage, because the moment you do, it will sap your strength and emerge victorious. The task is to get to know and befriend your fear. Use it as a warning mechanism and not as a trigger for the fight-or-flight response. My mentor used to tell me that fear was the absence of love. I was confused. I told him that the Amazon shamans, as part of their discipline, went into the jungle alone in the dark of the moon to meet their fear. The one time I had tried it, I emerged terrified. The hair at the back of my neck had stood on end the entire night. I believed I was being stalked by every large carnivore in the jungle and by all the haunting spirits of the place. The old man smiled. He said that this was an interesting enough practice, but that the real task for the shaman was to embrace fear. "When you understand that the jaguar you heard and the ghosts you sensed were in your mind, you can dispel them," he said. "And when you have emptied yourself of fear you can meet the jungle cat in person and know that it is no different from you, that you are both expressions of the same life force."

I have been a vegetarian for a long time, principally because I am not willing to eat anything I'm not willing to kill. (I have also found that eating red meat dulls my seeing abilities.) During my training with the Amazon shamans I was required to track, ceremonially kill, and then eat an animal whose power I sought to embody. The animal my teacher had selected for me to track was a water boa (*sachamama*), a magnificent brown and yellow creature that favored the shallow tributaries of the Amazon. While I did not have a hard-and-fast rule about not eating meat (I did so when the shamans I visited prepared it on some special occasion), for the longest time I refused to do this exercise. I even left the jungle and returned to the United States, thinking that if my training required taking the life of an animal, then I was not willing to continue. Yet something drew me back to the Amazon, and I decided to follow through at least with the tracking part of the exercise. I would see later about the killing and eating.

Boas can grow to enormous size, the largest stretching as much as twenty feet in length and weighing more than six hundred pounds. They are relatively easy to spot in the water or the land but difficult to track, as they are very cunning and can remain submerged for long periods of time.

I understood that the *sachamama* represented passion and sexuality as well as creativity and the ability to see beneath the surface of things. I had been tracking boas for several days, not managing to get close enough to one to take its picture, when out of sheer frustration I sat down by the edge of the river. I pulled out a bag of trail mix and contemplated the water flowing soundlessly by. I asked myself why I had such a reluctance to kill for food. I was genuinely repulsed at the thought of killing an animal as beautiful as a water boa. In my reverie, I began to reflect on the love with which a jaguar snaps the neck of a deer it will eat. There was no malice associated with this act. I suddenly realized that my killing a water boa was violent only because I considered myself separate from this grand snake. As long as we were disjoined, eating it would simply extinguish its life to provide me with food, and therefore it would be an act of violence.

It dawned on me that the snake and I were manifestations of the same life force. We were not different. It was life feeding on itself. The snake would continue to live within me, and in that instant both of us would become part of a much greater force. I snapped out of my reverie, and my gaze wandered to a nearby bush, to light reflecting from a scale. It was a seven-foot-long water boa that had just feasted on some large rodent and was in a reverie similar to mine. I couldn't believe my eyes. The snake lay coiled, digesting its meal, with a large bulge about a foot into its body. A snake this size eats only once every few weeks. After a meal it becomes sluggish. While it digests its food, it cannot move. Here was the answer to my quest.

I picked up the serpent, which wrapped itself lazily around my arms and shoulders. I walked back to the shaman's hut and proudly showed her the coiled snake. She began to laugh, and continued chuckling for several minutes. I was beginning to get annoyed. I asked her why I needed to eat the boa to receive the gift of its power. The old woman smiled and said that knowledge was not easily absorbed through the digestive tract. She grinned and told me to find a protected place near the water where the snake would be out of harm's way. With time I discovered that violence was something I had to conquer within me, not outside myself by making rules about what I could or could not eat. I had learned the lessons I came for.

Second-chakra personality disorders can take a high toll. These people live in a world where the rain falls because the sky personally wants to get them wet. At times they believe the entire world is conspiring against them. Granted, sometimes it does rain for us, but it also rains for the trees, plants, animals and stones, as well as for its own sake. This person often has an attitude of entitlement. As he heals his second chakra he discovers that the world owes him nothing. On the contrary, he has a debt to life. Under the direction of the second chakra, the center of erotic love, we explore our passion and discover intimacy. Dysfunction in this chakra can lead one to confuse sex with love. The great task of the second chakra is to transform sex into love, romance into intimacy. This is no easy task, as the negative drives of this chakra are a need to control others through money, power, and sex. The second chakra passes right though the womb, where life germinates. This center germinates the seeds of passion and creativity that will bloom in our upper chakras.

THE THIRD CHAKRA

ELEMENT: Fire

COLOR: Yellow

BODY ASPECTS: Stomach, abdomen, liver, pancreas, storing and releasing energy, spleen

INSTINCT: Power

PSYCHOLOGICAL ASPECTS: Courage, power, expression in the world

GLAND: Pancreas

SEEDS: Autonomy, individuation, selfless service, fulfillment of dreams, longevity

NEGATIVE EXPRESSIONS: Gastrointestinal disorders, anorexia, sorrow, pride, ego inflation, neurotic symptoms, low energy, victim mentality, temper tantrums, shame

The third chakra is located at the solar plexus and is associated with the pancreas. This gland is the energy banker of the body. Glucose is its currency. (The pancreas manufactures insulin, which gets glucose from the bloodstream into the cells, where it can be used for fuel.) When the third chakra is functioning properly, the body has plentiful energy for all its activities. Since the brain is the largest fuel consumer in the body, a balanced third chakra is essential for clear thinking. It also influences the liver, which is the fuel storehouse of the body. Individuals with third-chakra disorders often suffer from low energy. The foods they eat are eliminated before their nutrients reach the bloodstream. Problems with sustenance may appear on the psychological and spiritual levels. When the third chakra is not functioning properly, a person will fail at his endeavors. Even though he has all the resources for success at hand, he does not have the stamina to get to the finish line.

The third chakra is the power center in the luminous energy system. Its power can be used constructively, to manifest our aspirations in the world. When used destructively, it can repress our primary nature or libido, which manifests as neurotic symptoms including shame and guilt. This chakra corresponds chronologically to the ages of fourteen to twenty-one, the years that precede adulthood.

The feminine power of the first chakra and the primordial sexual energy of the second chakra are transformed into a fine fuel that the third chakra employs for the fulfillment of our dreams. This chakra replenishes the reserves in the Luminous Energy Field. When we awaken the power of this chakra, we experience fearlessness and a resolve that cannot be deterred by adversity. Obstacles in our path crumble. The danger is that this can result in ego aggrandizement. We begin to think that we are the sole authors of our destiny and can subject the world to our will. We feel capable of creating or destroying the world and become dictatorial and manipulative, striving for personal power and fame at whatever cost. Individuals seduced by the power of the third chakra often seek to control others through intimidation. When this chakra is cleared, our family and interpersonal relationships become stable. We become effective communicators and discover the power of the spoken and written word. This center makes us true to our own nature. Our life purpose becomes clear, and we can align ourselves to it.

There are stories of Inka warriors whose third chakra shone like a golden disk. Legend says they could not be killed. The conquistadors would fire their muskets at them, but the bullets would always miss their mark. There are similar legends among the Plains Indians in

North America, of braves the cavalry would shoot at but never hit. The Inka lore tells us that when one of these luminous warriors slayed an adversary, he would honor the other by shedding a few drops of his own blood into the earth. He realized that in other circumstances they might have been sitting together exchanging stories around the fire. These men and women believed that you were already dead if you went into battle angry or afraid.

When I was writing *Dance of the Four Winds*, I went to Rio de Janeiro with my coauthor for a couple of weeks of undisturbed work. I had just completed an expedition to the Amazon, and a friend had offered me his apartment on the beach in Rio. On our final evening, after a celebratory dinner, we were walking back along the beach to our apartment when we were attacked by six men. As we grappled with the muggers time seemed to slow down, and I suddenly understood the teachings of the luminous warriors. I stopped fighting and shouted, "Halt!" The yell seemed to pierce the night, and everyone stopped. I turned to the ringleader and offered him my watch, saying that he had to change the batteries every two years. Then I gave him my wallet. I turned to another and asked him his shoe size. He replied that it was 44. I said that this was my exact size and asked him to try on my shoes. They fit him well and a smile came over him. Eric, my coauthor, could not believe his eyes, and began struggling again. Immediately three of the men wrestled him down on the sand. I walked over to Eric and explained to him that these men were poor, that they needed our watches, wallets, shoes, and belts. At the end of the exchange the ringleader shook my hand, and then each of the other thieves thanked us. I waved and wished them well. As we parted, I asked the leader if he had a car. He said no, and then I mentioned that he probably would not need my driver's license. He smiled and said of course not and handed it back to me. He couldn't use my credit cards either, he said, and gave those back. Then he returned my passport and travel documents. Eric was stunned. The thieves were giving us back our belongings. While we were still robbed, we were not violated. We practiced nonviolence and so were able to change the entire tone of the encounter. We tempered a second-chakra negative reaction and responded from the third chakra.

The function of the third chakra is to translate vision into reality. The name of this chakra in Sanskrit is *manipura*, which means "the palace of jewels," referring to its ability to transform dreams into living treasures. The shaman understands that you dream the world into being. This center is the alembic on which our dreams are alchemically turned into gold. When you want to improve the world around you, bring balance to your third chakra. The tool of this center is visualization — whether sitting in meditation or on your feet at the beach being mugged. The fire element that rules it provides the fuel to manifest dreams. Be careful that you do not exercise this power for personal gain, but rather for the common good. The key word for this chakra is *service*.

THE FOURTH CHAKRA

ELEMENT: Air

COLOR: Green

BODY ASPECTS: Circulatory system, lungs, breasts, heart, asthma, immune deficiencies

INSTINCT: Love

PSYCHOLOGICAL ASPECTS: Love, hope, surrender to another, compassion, intimacy

GLAND: Thymus

SEEDS: Selfless love, forgiveness

NEGATIVE EXPRESSIONS: Ego aggrandizement, resentment, selfishness, grief, loneliness, abandonment, betrayal

The heart chakra is located at the cardiac plexus, in the center of the chest, not over the heart itself. It is the axis of the chakra system. Just as the belly is at the center of gravity of the physical body, the heart is at the center of the luminous body. The thymus gland is regulated by the heart chakra. The thymus is responsible for cell-mediated immunity. It is one of the main players in the immune response, critical in the development of B and T lymphocytes, the body's "killer cells." Persons with a depressed immune system respond excellently when the heart chakra is cleared through the Illumination Process.

The Sanskrit name for the heart chakra is *anahata*, which means "unbound." It refers to how we become free from the material measures of success. Money, automobiles, fame, and fortune cease being the measures of achievement. Freedom, joyfulness, and an abiding peace become the hallmarks of a person who dwells in his heart center. Chronologically, the heart chakra is associated with the ages of twenty-one to twenty-eight. It is the center from which we form our families and discover love with our soul partners and our children.

Through the heart center we share and experience love. This is the most misunderstood chakra in the body, because the quality of love of the heart chakra is neither the affection that we exchange with each other nor the romantic love we "fall" into. The heart chakra thrives on the love of Creation, the same love that the flowers feel for the rain or that the jaguar feels for the antelope it will have for a meal. This kind of love is not object-focused, nor is it dependent on another for its existence. It is not sentimental. It is impersonal. Christian theologians call it *agape*. The Inka call it *munay*. This kind of love is not a means to an end. It does not lead to marriage or relationships. It is an end in itself.

While traveling through the Andes several years ago, my companions and I were caught in a blizzard. We were accompanying an Indian woman who was taking her three-month-old baby to a clinic in the valley below. We took refuge in an abandoned hut that protected us from the snow and hail, yet the wind howled mercilessly through the gaps in the stone wall. We huddled together while María held the baby close to her chest. All during the night, the mother attempted to nurse the child, opening her blouse and bringing the baby's lips to her breast. By morning the storm had subsided, and the hills were covered with a blanket of white. As the dawn broke we all stepped outside to warm ourselves in the sun. When María unbundled her baby, we discovered that the girl had died sometime during the night. We returned to the village, where a medicine woman blessed the baby and performed the death rites. I then accompanied the young mother into the hills and attempted to console her as we dug a shallow grave in the frozen ground. Both of us were in tears, and we said a prayer to Pachamama, Mother Earth, to receive her child. When we were done, we covered the mound with a pile of stones and returned to the village.

Two days later María was back working in her family's fields. They were turning over the soil to prepare the ground for planting. I was still distraught and had spent the previous days grieving the baby's death. When María saw how upset I was, she came over, hugged me, and said, "Do not be sad. My baby is now back with her mother." Her comment cut right through my anguish. I walked to the glacial stream at the edge of the village, stripped down to my shorts, and waded into the shallows. The frigid water shocked me out of my self-indulgent sentimentality. María then led me to the medicine woman who had performed her child's death rites. The old woman pressed her hand against my heart and with a kind look said to me that there was nothing to be sad about. I could hardly believe it. She was trying to comfort me. Later that evening, her family thanked me for accompanying María through that long, numbingly cold night. Though visibly sad, they were filled with warmth and compassion. I had never known a selfless love like this before. Egotism, no matter how altruistic it might seem, can create terrible imbalances in the fourth chakra.

To experience selfless love we must die to who we have been in the past. Thus shamans have devised intricate practices for experiencing the death of the ego and egotism. However, we do not need to go through the complicated death rites of the jungle shamans to experience the love of the heart chakra. We simply need to surrender to love — to translate love from a feeling into a practice and a meditation. We need to stop falling in love and become love itself. When you experience your heart beating, remind yourself that it is love that is beating.

One of the negative expressions of this chakra is an infatuation with the self. We all know people who claim to know that "love is the answer," who spout all the right clichés about love. These individuals are more interested in demonstrating their "enlightenment" than in practicing charity or selfless love. Another negative expression of our love instinct is the inability to show compassion for ourselves. When self-love is absent, we become stuck in self-criticism and shame. An impaired heart chakra makes us unable to commit to an intimate relationship. This person will run away at the moment she feels vulnerable, often using work or other distractions to keep herself from her beloved. A balanced heart chakra allows us to commit to intimacy in love. It integrates the masculine and feminine principles within us, and we no longer seek our "missing half" outside ourselves. Soft and hard, receptivity and creativity cease to be opposites, as these principles are joined in a delicate harmony. The heart center allows us to recover an innocence that makes us playful and inspired. We know who we are and we accept ourselves, which brings us joy and peace.

THE FIFTH CHAKRA

ELEMENT: Light

COLOR: Blue

BODY ASPECTS: Throat, mouth, neck, esophagus

INSTINCT: Psychic expression

PSYCHOLOGICAL ASPECTS: Manifesting dreams, creativity, communication, faith

GLANDS: Thyroid, parathyroid

SEEDS: Personal power, faith, will

NEGATIVE EXPRESSION: Betrayal, addictions, psychosis, sleep
   disorders, lies, fear of speaking out, gossiping, toxicity

The fifth chakra is located at the hollow of the throat and influences the thyroid gland, the temperature regulator in the body. By regulating the rate of metabolism, that is, the rate at which fuel is burned in the body, it affects body weight and the replenishment of vitamins. The Sanskrit name for this chakra is *vishuda,* which means "purity." The most ancient of all yogic texts, inscribed fifteen hundred years ago by Patanjali, speaks about the *siddhis* or magical powers available to someone who has awakened this luminous center. These powers include the ability to bilocate, to become invisible, to look into the past, and to discern the workings of destiny.

The fifth chakra is our psychic center, responsible for clairvoyance, clairaudience, clairsentience, and the ability to communicate without words. A dysfunctional fifth chakra can result in unwanted psychic experiences, even in a borderline personality who is easily susceptible to psychosis and neurosis. His fantasies involuntarily spill into his everyday world, and he cannot distinguish fantasy from reality. Sleep disorders are common when this chakra is out of balance.

Chronologically, the fifth chakra corresponds to the ages of twenty-eight to thirty-five, when we begin to make our mark in the world. When the fifth chakra is clear, we begin to achieve recognition in our fields of endeavor and acquire mastery in our chosen profession. Our experience and knowledge define our status in the world. The fifth chakra gives us the ability to envision possible futures and to act on our vision. You imagine who you can become and feel the freedom of infinite possibilities. In this center true introspection becomes possible as the fullness of our interior world becomes available to us for the first time. The fifth chakra allows us to look within, to become aware of our inner processes. We develop a vocabulary for our emotional, psychological, and spiritual life. This spiritual vocabulary will grow in breadth and scope in our sixth chakra, together with the ability to look for inner resources anytime we feel we need to change the outside world. In the fifth chakra we begin to develop a global perspective. We no longer fixate only on our group, tribe, or culture. We begin to identify with all peoples regardless of race or birthplace. In the first chakra we derive our identity from our mothers; in the second it comes from our families; in the third chakra we rebel against our parents and identify with our peer group; in the fourth we identify with our nation or culture (pop or otherwise). In the fifth chakra we become planetary citizens.

The fifth chakra gives voice to the feelings of the heart. It speaks out our love, kindness, and forgiveness. In this center the four elements — earth, water, fire, and air — of the lower chakras are combined into pure energy, which provides the matrix or framework for our dreams, like the honeycomb that gives form to a bee's hive. The throat chakra deploys this matrix around which we create our world.

An awakened throat chakra brings us into synchronicity with life. We've all had mornings when we wonder if we should have simply stayed in bed, when everything seems to be working against us. You go into the kitchen and discover that there is no cereal left; you get into your car and hit all the red lights on your way to work. When the universe turns adversarial, when things are out of sync, we can bring ourselves back into a synchronous relationship with life by clearing the throat chakra and dispelling the debris and dense energies that clutter it. The fifth chakra acts like a smokestack for all the lower centers, releasing the volatile energies that are not mulched into the Earth by the first chakra. A simple way to clear the throat chakra is to tap it three times with your fingertips. I do this several times during the day, especially after I have worked with a very "toxic" client.

A negative expression of this chakra is the intoxication with your own knowledge. These people do not listen to others in a conversation. Being right is more important than being understanding. The danger of the fifth chakra is its tendency to turn spiritual insight into dogma. This fifth-chakra pathology has affected nations and churches, as evidenced by the Inquisition and the religious intolerance in the world today.

For ordinary persons the fifth chakra serves as a smokestack to discharge energies combusted by the lower chakras. Most people use their voice nearly exclusively to communicate the emotional needs of their lower chakras. As we become conscious of our psychological and spiritual resources, this chakra grows in strength. We discover our true voice.

SKY CHAKRAS

In the sixth, seventh, eighth, and ninth chakras development becomes transpersonal. We explore increasingly subtle domains. Here is where we get into trouble. New Age ascension spirituality furthers the notion of an otherworldly God above and overlooks the practical spirituality of the feminine Earth. The sky chakras are supported by the Earth chakras, just as the branches of a tree are supported by its roots. The gifts of the higher chakras are immensely practical and manifest in *this* world. They are not otherworldly. This truth has been recognized by every great spiritual teacher. When Christ taught that "the kingdom of Heaven is at hand," he implied that Heaven and Earth are one, indivisible.

We are familiar with Earth-chakra issues from psychotherapy and our personal growth. We've all had to deal with mommy and daddy issues, with anger, shame, fear, sex, desire, and the longing for safety. In the sky chakras we enter into less familiar territory. These chakras hold attributes that are sometimes difficult to grasp. In some cases the distinction between the attributes of two chakras will be only a matter of degree. Think of the love a child feels for his mother versus the love he later feels for his beloved. While they both fall under the category of love, they are distinctly different experiences (despite what psychology would have us believe — that people generally end up marrying their opposite-sex parent). So it is with the spiritual lessons and attributes of the higher chakras.

When my mentor and I were mapping the domains of the sky chakras, we identified attributes that corresponded to these centers. Stepping beyond death was the attribute of the sixth chakra; mastery of time was the attribute of the seventh; invisibility the attribute of the eighth; and the ability to keep a secret was the attribute of the ninth.

THE SIXTH CHAKRA

ELEMENT: Pure light

COLOR: Indigo

BODY ASPECTS: Brain, eyes, nervous system

INSTINCT: Truth

PSYCHOLOGICAL ASPECTS: Reason and logic, intelligence, empathy, depression, stress-related disorders, denial

GLAND: Pituitary

SEED: Enlightenment, self-realization

NEGATIVE EXPRESSION: Delusion, neuroses, inadequacy, seizures

The sixth chakra, or third eye, is located in the middle of the forehead. In the Hindu traditions it is thought to be the third eye of Shiva, who grants knowledge of perfect truth and nonduality. The name of this center in Sanskrit is *ajna*, or "unlimited power." In this chakra we attain the knowledge that we are inseparable from God. We express the divine within ourselves, and we see the divine in others. We feel deep calm and peace when we are in the presence of one who has attained this realization. You realize that you are an eternal being inhabiting a temporal body. A person with an awakened sixth chakra realizes that the authentic self must shed its exclusive identification with bodily or mental experiences. We transcend body and mind, yet welcome both into the field of our awareness. As we begin to observe the mind, we can step into transpersonal states. We follow the mind with curiosity yet without being absorbed by it. Doubt disappears when you step beyond the mind, and desire and longing cease to be driving forces. One enters the realms of knowledge that can be experienced but not told. It is not that these realms lie outside the domain of words, but rather that experience is all there is. Shamans say that this is a realm that cannot be found through seeking, but that only those who seek may find it. It is like two lovers who no longer are separate but rather are united by a single kiss. When there is no experiencer, what can be said about the experience? The moment that it is told, it shatters. It is like waking from a dream. The moment we realize we were dreaming, the dream can no longer be remembered.

When the sixth chakra is malfunctioning, the individual confuses information with knowledge. He feels he has attained great spiritual truths when all he has is a collection of facts. Shamans know how to make it rain without being able to explain that water is made up of hydrogen and oxygen atoms. Spiritual materialism is an endemic dysfunction of the third-eye chakra. These individuals often exercise great power and influence in the world without assuming responsibility for its stewardship. In our media-driven world with its cult of celebrity, the energies of the sixth chakra can become distorted and result in spiritual arrogance and self-aggrandizement.

As an anthropologist, I have learned that every contact you have with an indigenous group corrupts the culture you are studying. The foods you bring with you, your camera and tools, and even your Western clothing are disruptive. The Inka that I had studied with, including Doña Laura and Don Manuel, still spun wool and made their own clothing by hand. They had none of the accoutrements of the West. Yet after witnessing the death of María's child, I let go of the anthropological maxim not to interfere. I began collecting children's clothing among our students to take to the Inka highlands. As a result of the many generous donations we received, we provided jackets and winter outfits for every child in six highland villages. In 1992 we began sending medical teams to assist the villagers. Although they had little contact with the West, they had become afflicted by the illnesses of civilization. We provided medical assistance to more than three hundred adults and children every year in a tent that served as a field clinic high up in the mountains. One year individuals who had read about our work traveled to these remote villages for a photo expedition and left behind a few boxes of baby formula, which several women then began to use in preference to nursing their babies. A few months later a mother came to us in our tent clinic and showed us her four-month-old child. She had run out of baby formula three weeks earlier, and her breast milk had dried up. The baby was skin and bones. He weighed less than eight pounds. We left her all of the infant food supplements we had, and encouraged her to allow one of her neighbors to nurse her child until the boy could begin eating solid foods. These well-meaning travelers had left dangerous gifts behind.

I've come to the realization that we have to discover the shaman within. I teach my students that no amount of traveling with the Indians will bring you to your own wisdom and power. I've found that it frequently achieves exactly the opposite, distracting us from a true encounter with Spirit. The shaman is a self-realized person. She discovers the ways of Spirit through her inner awakening. Antonio would remind me that the Buddha was not a Buddhist, and that Christ was not a Christian. One sat under a banyan tree until he gained illumination. The other went to the desert for forty days. In the sixth chakra we experience our own awakening. We shed the ponchos, the robes, the rattles and feathers, and all other exterior markings.

An awakened third eye allows the shaman to know who he is. It gives him knowledge of the past and future and allows him to envision alternative destinies. Some legends report that those who awaken this chakra can even attain physical immortality. They no longer age or succumb to disease, but rather are able to maintain their youthful vitality and strength. All the desires of one with an awakened third eye come true, and if a number of healers hold the same vision, it comes true for the planet. Native religions have long practiced this tradition. Elders of the Hopi and a similar council of Inka medicine men and women sit in meditation envisioning the kind of world that they want their great-grandchildren to inherit.

THE SEVENTH CHAKRA

ELEMENT: Pure energy

COLOR: Violet

BODY ASPECTS: Skin, brain, hormonal balances

INSTINCT: Universal ethics

PSYCHOLOGICAL ASPECTS: Selflessness, integrity, wisdom

GLAND: Pineal

SEEDS: Transcendence, illumination

NEGATIVE EXPRESSION: Psychoses, regression, cynicism

The crown chakra at the very top of the head is our portal to the Heavens, in the same way that the first chakra is the portal to the Earth. Luminous threads from this center reach up to the stars and to our destinies. The Earth protects us and nurtures us with her life force, and the Heavens propel us toward our becoming. Seeds sprout only when they are in the rich, dark, moist Earth, yet they grow by the light of the Sun. After germination, all plants turn to sunlight for life. Similarly, our spiritual life germinates in the first chakra with our nexus to the Earth, and later the light of the Heavens enters through the crown to feed the entire chakra system. The name for this chakra in Sanskrit is *sahasrara*, which means "emptiness." Persons who have attained the gifts from this center no longer need a physical form. Able to travel through space and time, they are one with Heaven and Earth.

The lesson of the seventh chakra is mastery of time. When we break free of linear, causal time, we are no longer in the tyrannical grip of the past. Today is no longer the result of an earlier incident, and we experience freedom from cause and effect. We live with one foot in the ordinary world and one foot in the spiritual world, and we realize that they share common ground. Whereas in the sixth chakra the healer acquires knowledge of past and future events, when she awakens the gifts of the seventh chakra she is able to influence those events. She can help heal events that happened in the past, and assist her client to select an alternative future, perhaps one in which the person is free of disease or leads a more fulfilling life.

In the seventh chakra the shaman is freed from desire, hope, or regret. On the upper Madre de Dios River, near the border between Peru and Brazil, lives an old medicine man, a master at working with the *ayahuasca*, a jungle potion that allows one, when properly guided, to experience the domains beyond death. This old man seldom speaks anymore — he has no use for words. During the ceremony he whistles and sings the songs of the river and the medicine plants, and you experience yourself as one with the rain forest around you. You and the river are no longer separate; the crickets, the cicadas, and you are all notes played by a single flute. In the seventh chakra we understand that life is an intricate web of luminous strands, and that each of us is one of these strands, but also that we are the entire web. I remember the first time I worked with this shaman. It had been more than five years since I had last taken the *ayahuasca*. I knew what to expect of this plant medicine, having tried it many times. Or so I thought. About an hour after ingesting the plant I had a vision of myself dying. I saw my body before me, lifeless, and observed it from a distance. I knew my identity was intact. I was the observer, not the corpse. Then the nausea hit me, and I ran outside into the jungle and got sick. Everything around me was pulsing and throbbing with life: the giant creepers, the hanging vines, the colossal trees that provide the canopy for all arboreal life. Everything was alive except me. I had become a living corpse, no longer the observer. I felt the pain of my life and the loss of my loved ones. I was stricken with grief. Then I became the observer again and felt free. For the next chunk of eternity I went back and forth between these two perspectives, pain and peace, bondage and freedom, life and death, until I understood that they were one and the same. In the seventh chakra there is no longer subject and object. Everything is participatory. Apparent contradictions are merged into one: life in death, peace in pain, freedom in bondage.

The negative expression of the seventh chakra is spiritual regression masquerading as enlightenment. Although it is true that in order to experience transcendence one must step beyond ego, we often think that every nonego state is transcendent. The belief that if you get rid of the ego you have Spirit is far from the truth. Many nonego states exist at different levels. For example, an infant's sense of self is undifferentiated from its surroundings. In psychotherapy, a lack of ego boundaries is recognized as unhealthy. The egos of people with severe mental illnesses, such as schizophrenia, are so fragmented that they are dysfunctional. In traditional cultures, the initiation process is carefully designed to make certain that the student has built a solid sense of himself before attempting to dismember the ego and attain this level.

In our culture of instant gratification spiritual seekers often want to leapfrog over the work of the lower chakras. Some seekers are lured by the promise of exotic experiences. Others are simply impatient or are not fully aware that they still have to clear their lower chakras in preparation for this work. Sometimes even their teachers have not completed this process and may not be aware themselves of its necessity. These individuals believe that whatever level of development they attain defines enlightenment, openly rejecting the suggestion that there is further to go. This kind of spiritual misconception is rampant today.

Those who have mastered the seventh chakra attain unusual powers, including remembering ancient memories belonging to the collective consciousness of humanity. Doña Laura used to tell me that the final test of the shaman who attempts this level is to remember the first story ever told.

"When time was still young, before the arrival of the four-leggeds or the plants, the first story ever told was told to us by the Stone People," she would say. "This is why we place a circle of stones around our fires."

I would implore her to tell me more.

"Ask the stones," she would say. Until one day I remembered.

Another gift of the seventh chakra is the ability to shape-shift. These shamans understand that they are no different from the stones, the plants, or the Earth. Laura once appeared in one of our meetings as a beautiful young Indian woman. I was very drawn to her and became enamored of her eyes and her smile. At one moment during the evening she went behind a boulder, and the person who returned an instant later was Doña Laura, one of the homeliest people I have ever met.

"You don't think I'm pretty anymore?" she asked, smiling.

Individuals who master the gifts of this chakra understand that the river of life flows beyond form and formlessness, beyond existence and nonexistence. They know infinity independent of time or form.

THE EIGHTH CHAKRA

ELEMENT: Soul

COLOR: Gold

BODY ASPECTS: Architect of the body

INSTINCT: Transcendence

PSYCHOLOGICAL ASPECTS: None

GLAND: None

SℰℰDS: Timelessness

Nℰgativℰ ℰxprℰssion: Templates of disease, cosmic horror

Don Antonio called the eighth chakra the *wiracocha*, or "source of the sacred." This might have been his unique way of describing this center, for I have not heard other medicine people call it such. This chakra resides a few inches above the head, and when awakened shines like a radiant sun inside the Luminous Energy Field. When a person shifts his awareness to the eighth chakra, he can access ancestral memory. He recalls knowledge that he never experienced directly. For example, he spontaneously may remember sitting on the prairies around a fire with the buffalo behind him, or praying inside stone temples above the snow line. The teachings of all shamans who have lived before become available to him. Their voices become his voice, and these ancient teachers live within him. This center is linked to the archetypal domain, the original images and memories that belong to the human collective.

The information fields in the eighth chakra act as the template to create the physical body. This chakra is like a carpenter who builds a chair (the physical body) and later burns it in his fireplace. The carpenter feels no loss, as he knows that he can simply build another out of new wood. The eighth chakra is unaffected by the death of the body. If an imprint of disease exists in this chakra, it is like a design flaw that is replicated with each new chair.

In the eighth chakra we experience a deep union not only with all of Creation, which happens in the seventh chakra, but with the Creator. The Creator is ineffable and cannot be encapsulated into an image that can be held by our senses. These encounters are often culturally scripted. A Christian may experience the union with the Creator as a fusion with an angel, a saint, or Christ. A Buddhist may experience it as communion with the Buddha, and an Inka shaman as a fusion with our local star, the Sun. We become one with the Creator and perceive the archetypal faces of the divine that exist in this realm. These are the images of God that have been etched and carved and painted by our ancestors for a hundred thousand years.

The negative expression of this chakra is cosmic horror, such as is experienced by those caught between the worlds of spirit and matter. Neither living nor dead, they are trapped in a nightmarish realm they can't awaken from. On the spiritual dimension, this is purgatory, what the Buddhists call the *bardo* planes. Disincarnate entities who cling to people or places on the Earth are trapped in this domain. Persons who suffer a spontaneous yet unbalanced awakening of this center can also become stuck in this realm. Many are in mental institutions; others suffer alone in their homes. Still others join bizarre pseudomystical cults.

The attribute of the eighth chakra is invisibility. In this center we become aware of the Beholder (known in Buddhism as the Witness)—a self that has been present from the beginning of our spiritual journey. Now disengaged from the mind, it is able to behold the mind with all of its dramas without subscribing to them. The Beholder witnesses our life unfolding and understands that all of the stories we use to describe ourselves are only stories. Everything we think we know about ourselves is not the real self. The Beholder knows that anything that can be seen or held is not real. The Beholder cleaves to the mystery and not the manifestation. The Beholder perceives everything but cannot itself be perceived, because it cannot be turned into an object of perception. The Beholder is invisible because it cannot be beheld.

Once, while hiking along the bank of a river with a jungle medicine woman and her husband, we came to a clearing. They said to me, "Alberto, you walk ahead and notice what happens."

I took the first step back into the rain forest and noticed that it was full of song. The parrots were squawking, the monkeys chattering with each other, and other birds singing. By the third step all of the sounds of the jungle had come to a standstill. The medicine woman, who had been following me a few paces behind, drew near and said, "That's because they know that you have been kicked out of the Garden. That's why they've all stopped. They know that you have been cast out of paradise. You no longer talk to God."

I was convinced this was nonsense. A couple of hundred yards back we had passed two Shipebo Indians who were roasting a boa on a spit. I walked back and asked them if I could have some of the boa fat they had been collecting in a tin can. I was certain that the animals had smelled my deodorant or the toothpaste I had used that morning. I stripped to my shorts and smeared my body with boa fat, determined that I was going to smell like a snake slithering into the rain forest. I walked back into the jungle, and with the first step I took the music of the Amazon filled my ears. By the third step the jungle had fallen silent again.

Many years later, after I had learned the practice of invisibility, I was able to walk into the jungle and be recognized as belonging in the Garden, as someone who still spoke with nature. We achieve invisibility by eliminating the "me" projects, and through the practice of stillness.

Eventually the Beholder will begin to reveal its own source, which is Spirit, or the ninth chakra.

THE NINTH CHAKRA

Element: Spirit

Color: Translucent white light

Body aspects: None

Instinct: Liberation

Psychological aspects: None

Gland: None

Seeds: Infinity

Negative expression: None

The ninth chakra resides at the heart of the Universe. It is outside time and space; it extends through the vastness of space and connects to the eighth chakra by a luminous cord. The shaman can travel through this cord to experience the vast expanse of Creation. We call this center a chakra for lack of a better name. In reality it is the dwelling place of Spirit. It exists beyond the personal soul, which keeps us bound to the space-time continuum and salvation and which is associated with the eighth chakra. It is the spirit of every thing in the Universe. The Beholder turns out to be everything that is beheld.

The ninth chakra is the Self that has never been born and will never die. This Self is prior to time, and it never enters the river through which time flows. It is prior to space and existed before the Universe manifested. This is the self that never left the Garden of Eden.

The process of the ninth chakra is the ability to keep a secret, even from yourself. The secret is that a very long time ago that Immense Force that we know as God decided from Its place in the unmanifest void to experience Itself. So It manifested twelve billion years ago as a singularity from which all matter in our Universe was formed. The Immense Force continued to explore Itself through all forms of life, as grasshopper, whale, planets, and moons. Yet since the Immense Force was omnipresent and omniscient, each of Its manifestations also possessed these qualities. Therefore It had to keep the nature of Its being a secret even from Itself in order to know Itself through Its ten thousand forms.

When this center is awakened, there is a deep, rumbling laugh that echoes over the mountains and thunders across the sky.

CHAPTER 5

THE SHAMAN'S WAY OF SEEING

Nazca, site of giant etchings on the desert floor. They depict colossal hummingbirds, spiders, and geometric lines that extend to the horizon. Erich von Daniken called them landing fields for gods from outer space. Nothing could be further from the truth.

Shamans sketched enormous mandalas here to bring balance to Heaven and Earth. The rectangles, triangles, and lines are part of a sacred geometry now forgotten. But the power of these figures remains. Every time I enter the figures at night I am able to see energy. The moon has to be right. It's the eeriest thing. At first I perceive what looks like fingerprints hovering above the sand, which turn into figures. The strange thing is that we all see the same thing. Is this a group hallucination?

Last night the moon was right. A dozen of us worked at the edge of a gigantic spiral that lay like a coiled serpent on the desert. Eduardo explained that as we walked into the spiral we were shedding the past that haunted us. When we emerged from the spiral we summoned who we were becoming. When the shaman walked in I saw an opaque shape lurking behind him. I tapped Isabel on the shoulder. She is Doña Laura's oldest student and the best seer in the group.

"What is it?" I asked.

As Eduardo walked along the curve of the spiral he drew close to us. Then we saw it. It was the most hideous beast any of us could imagine, part reptile, part gorilla, part human. It was a *creature worthy of a Hieronymous Bosch painting. And it was gaining on Eduardo, grabbing him in its claws. And then it got swallowed by the Earth. Eduardo had reached the center of the spiral and had his arms outstretched to the Heavens.*

When he walked out we described what we had seen.

"That was La Chiconga," he said. "It's an elemental power animal that one of my maestros contrived a very long time ago. It was an unnatural being employed by sorcerers to harm people. When this maestro died, La Chiconga did not have another master, and came to me. I had not seen it in years. I'm happy that it is gone."

I knew that Eduardo had trained with sorcerers in his youth, before he undertook the way of the shaman healer. I had heard him speak of La Chiconga before, but thought it was only a story.

These energies can cling to you for a very long time.

JOURNALS

THE EXERCISES IN THIS CHAPTER DEVELOP YOUR ABILITY TO SEE energy. You will learn to sense the Luminous Energy Field, to perceive the rivers of light, and to read the swirling disks of the chakras. When you learn the shaman's way of seeing, you can track the original wound that caused an imprint in the Luminous Energy Field. It also allows you to track intrusive energies in the body and to detect and identify the presence of intrusive spirits that may be causing emotional or physical harm.

In my work with clients, I perceive a past traumatic event as if it were replaying itself before my eyes. Often the actual facts are not precise, but the theme and the emotional impact on my client are usually correct. With Diane, I perceived a young girl involved in an auto accident. She covered her head with her hands and shut her eyes tightly; her body became rigid, and then she left her physical body. The spirit seemed to hover above the girl and told me that she was not interested in coming back. It was not safe for her here. When I recounted this, Diane could not remember any accident; she had to ask her mother, who later confirmed that one had occurred when Diane was a child and that no one had been injured. Yet since then Diane had lived half in and half out of her body, never fully comfortable with herself, never feeling completely safe. Her Luminous Energy Field held this information intact.

Mayans, Hindus, Buddhists, Aborigines, Inkas, and early Christians have all portrayed the human energy field using the same lexicon of images. An artist decorating King Tut's tomb five thousand years ago in lower Egypt sketched the god Thoth with a luminous orb above his head, a moon glyph denoting his energy and ability to intercede with the cyclical nature of time. This halo is identical to the eighth chakra described by Amazon shamans. The jungle peoples believe the gifts of this chakra are exactly those represented by the mythical Egyptian god—the ability to step outside of time. Likewise, the halo of light depicted around Christ is essentially the same as the one portrayed encircling Buddha or around a Maori shaman in New Zealand. These images depicted in stone, in wood, and on canvas confirm the existence of seers who were able to perceive a numinous reality. These were not artists using the halo as a symbol only; they were seers. The similarity of their perceptions attest to an innate ability we all have to sense the human energy field.

While references to the Luminous Energy Field occur across the globe and throughout the ages, most Western thinkers still find the evidence difficult to accept. We believe that when Egyptian scribes, Dogon carvers, or Buddhist artisans drew a halo of light around their subjects they were making allegorical references to some other kind of enlightenment. We imagine this enlightenment as some inner state that saints and sages achieve. Because we usually cannot perceive it with our eyes, we are convinced it is not a literal fact. Moreover, science has not demonstrated the existence of the Luminous

Energy Field, so we do not believe it can be real. If we think about it, however, we realize that science hadn't measured gravity until Newton demonstrated that it was a fundamental law of nature, yet for thousands of years, apples fell from trees and water flowed downhill. Granted, gravity is easier to observe than the human energy field, but to shamans worldwide, the invisible world of energy and Spirit is as tangible as water flowing downhill.

Certain obstacles arise when Westerners embrace these shamanic practices. We live in a culture in which people who claim to see energies are dismissed as wacky or as downright unbalanced and in need of psychiatric attention. I remember such an incident when I was doing my psychology internship at a hospital in northern California. The day after I started working in the unit, a patient named Pietro came up to me and said: "I know who you are. You can't hide from me." He then began describing incidents from my childhood that no one outside my immediate family had any way of knowing. Pietro's psychic abilities had exploded open as a result of a bad LSD experience years earlier. He was in the psychiatric ward because he did not know how to shut off his seeing, and he went around alarming people with frightening personal observations. Our doctors and therapists often do not know how to help someone for whom these gifts emerge, whether frighteningly and abruptly, as for Pietro, or gently and spontaneously, as they sometimes do during childhood or adolescence. Pietro had to be kept heavily medicated, and there was no hope for a cure. In a tribal culture, he might have held a position assisting a shaman to diagnose disease.

The shaman's way of seeing is a talent that must be developed. In the same way that those with musical talent must practice and be encouraged in order to play an instrument skillfully, so must those who wish to see into the luminous world develop and refine this skill. For millennia, shamans around the globe perfected techniques for honing these skills. These techniques were developed in societies that bestowed great honor on people who were able to glimpse the invisible world. I have adapted the most valuable of these practices, which we teach our students in the Healing the Light Body School.

HOW WE SEE

Vision is a rather miraculous process that required millions of years of evolution to perfect. For many complex life forms — from grasshoppers to whales — it is the primary means of perception. Human vision relies on three components: the eyes; the optic nerve, and the visual cortex in the brain. The eyes convert light into electrical signals. These signals are carried by the optic nerve into the visual cortex, the "screening room" in the brain. The optic nerve transports a stream of electrons from the eyes to the brain in the same way that a television cable carries a signal to a TV set. The visual cortex, located behind the ears in the back of the head, then generates an image. All seeing, in effect, happens inside the head, although it appears that we see the world outside.

The eyes are of little use for perceiving the invisible world of energy and spirit. Our retinas register only a narrow band in the electromagnetic spectrum. They do not register infrared or ultraviolet, for example, which the skin readily responds to. The optic nerve does not help either, because it is a one-way cable that only connects the eyes to the screening room. The screening room, however, is an extraordinary structure. The visual cortex is able to translate energy (electrical impulses from the optic nerve) into living images. The mechanism for seeing energy is already in place. To perceive the Luminous Energy Field and the stories encoded within it, we need only to change the source of the signal and allow the visual cortex to do what nature designed it to do — to create images.

When your physician checks your heart, she might perform an electrocardiogram. The sensors attached to your chest send a signal through a wire to a chart recorder that shows the blips of your heartbeat. If she wanted to check the temperature of her wine cellar, she could simply attach a thermometer to the wall but still use the same recorder. With the right sensor and cable, the chart recorder can measure any type of activity, from heartbeats to earthquakes. With ordinary seeing, the eyes are the sensors, the optic nerve is the cable, and the visual cortex is the recorder. To see into the world of energy, we have to disengage the sensors (the eyes) and the cable (optic nerve), but we want to keep the recorder, the visual cortex. The sole function of the recorder is to translate a signal into an image. This is why I call it the screening room.

We have the sensors we need to develop the shaman's way of seeing—they are the sixth chakra (the mythic "third eye" in the center of the forehead) and the fourth chakra, the heart. By connecting the heart chakra and the third eye to the visual cortex, we can see with the eyes of the mind and the heart. The task is getting a "cable" from these chakras to the screening room in the back of the head.

As an anatomy student, I learned that the human brain is hardwired. After the neural pathways in the brain are established, it is very difficult to change them. It is impossible to lay new neurological tracks to the visual cortex. If the human optic nerve is severed, a person is blinded and does not recover vision. Yet he still dreams in full color and imagery. The brain cannot reroute the signals to the visual cortex. Thus, to see with the eyes of the heart, we must create an extracerebral network, outside the brain. The shaman's rites for seeing can lay extracerebral pathways that connect the heart and the third eye to the screening room of the visual cortex, to achieve multisensorial images of the luminous world.

For the first few years of life, babies have ten times the number of synaptic connections in their brain that adults have. Synapses are like branches that extend from nerve cells, forking in multiple directions, until they find another branch to link with. Synaptic connections are the pathways through which we process information. While we were toddlers we might have discovered six different ways to approach a water glass and pick it up. Eventually, as we learned the way that was best for us, including left- or right-handedness, the other pathways shriveled and died. Synapses connect one brain cell to another, and can be compared to trails in a forest. Some trails are very direct and lead one over grassland to the river. Other paths are more circuitous, through patches of poplars and elms, but eventually leading to the same river. Once we have drawn our maps of reality, 90 percent of our synaptic connections die. We become familiar with only one way to get to the river. The other routes are erased. If we learn the grassy path, we forget that poplars and birches exist. We look in disbelief at a traveler who tells of exotic trees he perceived on the way to the stream.

In our culture, mapping the landscape of the invisible world is not a priority. This spiritual landscape is not even acknowledged as real. There is no river, so why cut trails to get to it? Westerners have not developed the neural pathways to sense energy. So we must lay these pathways outside the brain. You can think of them as meridians of golden light routed along the outside of the head, connecting the third eye and the heart to the screening room in the back of the skull. These pathways relay multimodal sensory data — images, textures, sounds, tastes, feelings, and fragrances.

LOSING YOUR HEAD AND COMING TO YOUR SENSES

The invisible world cannot be seen with the eyes of logic and reason. We must resurrect the child's sense of innocence and rediscover primary, direct perception. A child explores textures, distinguishes colors, looks underneath stones, and asks the why of everything. This is immediate, primary perception. When Christ said, "Unless you be like a child you shall not enter the kingdom of Heaven," he is suggesting that we must learn to perceive the world again innocently, unencumbered by preconceptions. Language and reason separate us from direct experience. Names and logic, while practical, keep us from the mystery of life.

We want to engage the senses before practicing the exercises that follow. Otherwise the practice becomes an intellectual activity and limited to what the eyes can see. When we engage the senses we achieve a holistic perception of the world, so that touch, taste, hearing, and sight no longer separate us from experience, but make us one with what we perceive. You smell a fragrance and become the fragrance, indivisible from it. This is not a poetic kind of communion. It is a deep understanding of our interconnectedness. For example, when a medicine woman dips her cup into the headwaters of the Amazon, she doesn't think, *Ah, now this water is mine.* Instead she observes, *Now the Amazon flows through me.*

PERCEPTUAL EXERCISE

Take your pulse, but do not look at your watch. Don't count your heartbeat. Merely experience the tides that flow through you, the waves of lifeblood rushing within you. Feel the rhythm of your pulse. This is your tempo. No one else has a rhythm exactly like yours. Islanders in Indonesia believe that everything in life has a pulse. Thousands of years ago they cast bronze drums the size of an elephant and beat on them the rhythms of Creation to attune their spirit to the tempo of the Universe itself.

Use your imagination. What color is your blood? Are you sure it's red? Why is it that your veins are blue? When does your blood change color? Why? Don't think back to that biology class you had to take in high school. Your body knows the answer. Ask it. Follow your blood back to your heart and find the answer for yourself. The heart is the first organ to receive the red, oxygen-rich blood from the lungs, and it feeds itself first before pumping blood to feed the rest of the body.

Now bring your awareness to your breath. First cover one nostril and then the other. Which nostril are you breathing through? We breathe predominantly through one nostril for a few hours, and then the other. Follow your breath as it goes down your windpipe and into your lungs. What does it feel like? Does it sound raspy or smooth? Where did your breath come from, and how long is it yours?

Next engage your olfactory sense. What is your scent? Everyone has a unique scent. Smell your hand after you've chopped garlic or basil. Inhale many different scents: the sweet smell of flowers, the pungent smell of vinegar, the acrid smell of spoiled milk, the sweet scent of lavender. Most mammals rely first and foremost on their sense of smell. A polar bear is able to smell a seal thirty miles away. Monkeys sniff each other when they first meet. A lion in the bush will smell your fear.

After that, engage your sense of touch. The skin is the largest sensory organ in the body. It is fabricated from the same tissue as your brain and nervous system. Skin is alive. It erupts when it is angry, glows when it is pampered. Take a moment to caress your face. Feel your lips, passing your fingertips over their entire circumference. Caress the face of your beloved. Next, become aware of your feet. Wiggle your toes inside your shoes. The human brain works by inhibition. When you put on your shoes in the morning you are aware of the temperature and feel of the inside of your shoes. But then the brain inhibits this sensation, because, after all, you don't want to have to be aware of your shoes all day. Only if you bump against a chair or step on a tack do you again become aware of your feet. Next time you sit down to eat a meal, switch the hand you use to hold the fork and knife. Notice how awkward it feels, and use this sensation to become aware of every bite you take and the flavor of your food.

Engage your sense of taste. What does your skin taste like? Lick your forearm. Is it salty or sweet? What does your blood taste like? Try it next time you cut yourself, and be aware of the taste. What does water taste like? It is commonly held that tap water is tasteless. This is not true. Water has its own taste, and the water in every city and stream tastes different. Drink slowly and savor it. Feel the coolness of the water and become that coolness; feel it suffusing the entirety of your mouth and from there radiating through your body. Allow the coolness to fill you.

Finally, close your eyes, take a deep breath, and listen. What are the sounds around you? Try to identify as many natural sounds as you can. Is there a bird singing? Are there bees humming? Are the sounds around you all man-made? Is there anything rumbling? Any high-pitched squeaks or cries? When tracking jaguars in the Amazon you listen to the birds. Their warning cries alert you to the whereabouts of the big cats long before their tracks are visible.

To practice primary perception shamans have developed a kind of "common sense" that bridges all of the senses. They are able to taste fire, to touch the fragrance of a flower, and to smell an image. They attain immediate perception before an experience is divided among the senses, an ability known as synesthesia. This blending of sensory modalities seems strange only to those who have distanced them-selves from a direct, primordial experience of the natural world. Musicians often report hearing the air rushing past wing feathers as they observe birds in flight. This "common sense," which is the hall-mark of primary perception, is an ability that most of us have lost with the rise of civilization. As the philosopher Maurice Merleau-Ponty wrote in *Phenomenology of Perception*, "Synesthetic perception is the rule, and we are unaware of it only because scientific knowledge shifts the center of gravity of experience, so that we have unlearned how to see, hear, and generally speaking, feel, in order to deduce, from our bodily organization, the world as the physicist conceives it, what we are to see, hear and feel." Synesthesia grows as we bring awareness to touch, taste, sensation, and sound.

One of my favorite synesthesia exercises involves "tasting" your emotions. Become aware of the taste in your mouth. Is it sweet? Sour? Woody? Metallic? Now recall an incident that made you feel sad. Notice if the taste in your mouth changes. Recall a pleasurable situation, and notice again how the taste in your mouth changes.

Now recall an instance where you felt fear. Can you savor the taste of fear? Of love? Of joy?

THE SECOND ATTENTION EXERCISE

The Second Attention practice is an eye movement exercise that seems to recalibrate our neural networks. It resets our sensory coordinates to zero, so to speak, in less than thirty seconds. Otherwise our sensory perception remains locked into the first attention, the tunnel vision of ordinary reality. In this initial exercise, we will use the Second Attention practice to free our kinesthetic sense and perceive the acupuncture meridians. Once you can feel energy, you can translate this sensation into an image through synesthesia.

Imagine that your eyes are the face of a clock. The eyes act like a pointing device and signal the region of our brain we employ for different mental activity. For example, many right-handed people look toward ten o'clock when performing mathematical computations and toward two o'clock when recalling their favorite songs. Check this out with a coworker. Ask them to add twenty-seven plus nineteen, then observe in which direction they turn their eyes. Everyone responds differently, yet their eyes always point in the same direction every time. Now ask them to recall the smell of freshly baked bread, or a song. Observe which direction their eyes point toward. These are the perceptual coordinates of the first attention, of ordinary reality.

The Second Attention practice involves rotating your eyes with your eyelids shut, to clear the perceptual screen. Close your eyes and move them (without moving your head) from left to right, up to down, upper left to lower right, and vice versa. Now rotate your eyes in a big circle, left to right three times and then right to left three times. Repeat once more, rotating your eyes in small circles, eyelids shut.

Bring your hands together in the prayer pose. (The ten principal acupuncture meridians run throughout the body, passing through the hands and fingertips, and when we bring our hands together in a prayer pose we balance the energies that flow through the acupuncture meridians. Perhaps this is why this posture is associated with prayer, as we long to be in balance when we pray.) Be sure that there is a little space between the fingers of each hand and that the fingertips are touching each other, index to index, thumb to thumb, and so forth. Your hands should be resting gently against your chest. Take a few deep breaths while holding your hands together.

Next, separate your hands and shake them vigorously from side to side for about thirty seconds, relaxing and allowing them to become limp. Bring your hands together again in the prayer pose. Gradually separate your palms, keeping your fingertips together. Be aware of the feeling in your hands. Do they feel cool? Warm? Do you sense a slight electrical sensation between your palms? Separate your hands slowly, remaining aware of your fingertips. Do you feel tingling in the pads at the tips of your fingers? See how far you can separate your fingers and still maintain that tingling or electrical sensation. Imagine that you can sense the luminous threads that connect your fingertips to each other. These are extensions of the acupuncture meridians. Practice this a few times until you can sense your meridians with your hands twelve inches apart. Notice which hand is more sensitive. Can you sense the energy better with you left or your right fingertips?

SENSING THE LUMINOUS ENERGY FIELD

Next we want to learn to scan the membrane of the Luminous Energy Field. In a standing position, close your eyes and do the Second Attention practice. Become aware of your breathing. Zen meditators attend to the breath to keep the rational mind engaged while they explore other domains with their awareness.

Shake your hands vigorously for a few seconds and bring them together in the prayer pose. Slowly turn your hands so that your palms are facing out, away from the body. Gradually fan out your hands until they are about a foot away from your belly. Move your hands back and forth slowly, as if you were wiping a window clean, and try to sense the inner membrane or skin of the Luminous Energy Field. Is it smooth, or does it have a texture? Is it elastic, does it yield, or is it firm? Does it feel warm or cool? Can you push it out and expand it? (In the city the Luminous Energy Field is drawn tightly around us like a silk cocoon, while after a few days in nature it expands to the width of our outstretched arms.) Are there ridges and pockets in it? These usually indicate places where our luminous membrane is weak and where we leak energy or can be penetrated by energies and emotions belonging to others. Imagine the color of your Luminous Energy Field.

When you're done, return your hands to prayer pose for a few breaths to balance your energy. Practice this exercise until you are able to clearly sense the texture and feel of the membrane of your Luminous Energy Field.

READING THE CHAKRAS

We will use a similar exercise to sense the chakras. In this exercise we will work with the each of the Earth chakras. Repeat the Second Attention practice; shake your hands vigorously for a few seconds and bring them to prayer pose. Remain mindful of your breath.

Now bring the palms of your open hands about three inches below your navel, very close to your skin. Stay with your breath. Imagine your chakras as funnels of energy, spinning just outside your skin like whirlpools of light. The outer lip of the funnel lies three to four inches outside the body, while much of the length of the chakra resides within the body. Find the outer edge of the funnel of your second chakra. Sense its circumference and the energy whirling within it. When I place a finger in a chakra I sense the energy like cool water swirling past my fingertip.

Gradually bring your index finger into the chakra, going in toward the body. What does it feel like? Is it cool, warm, or neutral? Bring your attention to the very tip of your finger and sense what you feel on the pad. Is it tingly, soft, or rough? The belly chakra is associated with the fight-or-flight response. When we experience fear or danger, we immediately register it in this chakra. While you explore your second chakra with the tip of your finger, recall when you last felt afraid. Do you notice a difference in the feel and texture? Everyone senses energy differently. What you register as icy someone else might sense as warm. The second chakra is the easiest to read, as it is the seat of our passions and emotions, and holds a high charge. Repeat the exercise with the first chakra. Notice if the texture and density of the chakra changes when you recall a time when you felt safe and protected, perhaps when you were young. Now recall a time when you did not feel safe, or when you woke up from a nightmare. How is the energy different?

Now try sensing the third chakra. Recall a time when you were acknowledged and recognized for an achievement. Does the texture of the energy seem to change? Recall a time you felt ashamed. Now move up to the fourth chakra. Recall when you were in love, when you first met your spouse or partner. Now recall a time you felt abandoned or heartbroken. Notice the changes in the quality of the energy. Next try sensing the fifth chakra. Recall a time when you experienced great inner peace, perhaps during meditation. Now recall a time you felt you were not heard by a loved one. How is the energy different?

Until now, we have been working with quantitative measures. The exercises you've done thus far give you a sense of the texture and intensity of the energy in the chakras. Most healers do not get beyond this stage. They feel the strength and weakness of the energy and nothing more. We want to develop the next stage, the qualitative measures. What information does the energy contain? What are the stories, the joy and the pain? We achieve this through the Second Awareness. The Second Attention practice frees your sensory systems.

The Second Awareness allows you to read the stories contained in energy.

THE SECOND AWARENESS EXERCISE

The Second Awareness allows you to perceive the stories contained within energy. You install fibers of light along the scalp that relay information from the third eye to the visual cortex, where it can be decoded and displayed in vibrant color. We add to that the information streaming in from the heart on similar fibers of light. These extracerebral pathways convey emotional and spiritual insight. The third eye registers facts, while the heart registers feelings. In this way, your seeing is tempered by compassion. On its own, the third eye is cold and dispassionate. By itself, the heart gets gushy and sentimental. Working together, the two become the healer's most powerful sources of knowledge. Ninety percent of my students are capable of developing this skill. It is not a gift that only a select few are born with. The visual cortex is capable of envisioning anything. More than that, it decodes the information, deciphering images laden with symbols and meaning.

Assume the prayer pose and go through the Second Attention practice while taking several deep breaths. Next, with the fingertips of both hands tap the center of your chest at the level of your heart. Tap the outline of an imaginary necklace of light going from your heart chakra to the back of your skull, to the visual cortex. Repeat this movement slowly and mindfully three or four times.

Next tap on your sixth chakra, on the center of your forehead. Pat an imaginary band from your forehead to the base of your skull in the back of the head. Follow a line just above each ear. Repeat several times.

Now tap once again on your sixth chakra and follow a band along the top of your head (tapping with both hands along the midline) to the base of the skull. Imagine that you are placing a crown of light over your head.

CROWN OF LIGHT

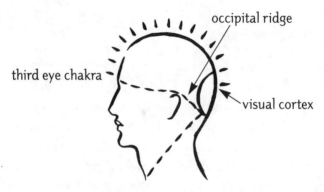

Tap along the dots.

NECKLACE OF LIGHT

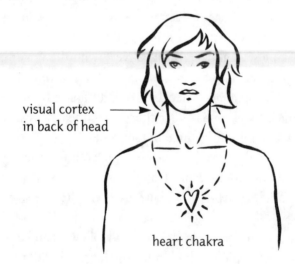

Tap along the dots.

As you visualize this crown and necklace, you install extracerebral pathways to the visual cortex of the brain. Visualize energy running through these pathways to activate them. I visualize these pathways as shimmering fibers and imagine a golden light streaming through them, slowly at first, then picking up speed and intensity until the entire network is pulsing with light. I have found that some students very quickly develop the ability to see. Their luminous pathways are readily installed and begin transmitting information right away. For others it can take months or even years. The Second Awareness cannot be achieved through trying, which is an act of the will and belongs in the world of our ordinary (first) awareness. Energize the extracerebral pathways and let the visual cortex of the brain do what it was designed to do.

You may realize one day that you have already been seeing for some time. It took me many months of practice, energizing the luminous pathways from my forehead and my heart to the back of my head, to achieve reliable results. One day I discovered that I had been seeing the Luminous Energy Field for months but simply had not been aware of perceiving it. It was a strangely familiar sensation. At first I could see the Luminous Energy Field and the chakras only with my eyes closed. I would bring my hands into prayer pose, breathe deeply, and observe the energy streams as I moved my fingers apart. Then I could focus my attention on a client and perceive her luminous body. At first ordinary sight was intrusive and distracting. With time I have learned to see with my eyes open as well. I employ the Second Awareness only after obtaining a client's permission (or before I board an airplane, to make sure everyone around me has a healthy Luminous Energy Field, a sure indication we will arrive safely).

Practice seeing the energy field around plants and animals. Notice the filaments that extend from a pet to its owner, or from your house-plants to nature and to your own Luminous Energy Field. The recognition that we can see the world of energy and spirit is the greatest validation not only of your ability, but of the reality of the invisible world.

Susan was in her early fifties when she enrolled in our Healing the Light Body School. A university professor, she had traveled with me to Peru nearly ten years earlier. We hadn't seen each other in several years. In the course of our conversation, she told me that she was experiencing incapacitating migraines on a daily basis. When the migraines came she was unable to teach, or even to walk, for nearly one hour. Her doctors had found nothing physically wrong with her, yet the migraines persisted. She asked if I would scan her Luminous Energy Field to sense what might be causing her headaches.

Susan sat against a white wall across from me. I dimmed the lights in the room. Softening my gaze, I brought my hands into prayer pose and entered into the calm state I have learned to associate with the Second Awareness. I immediately sensed that Susan's seventh chakra was blocked. No energy flowed in or out of this area. Ordinarily the seventh chakra is like a fountain of energy gushing out the top of the head and streaming through the Luminous Energy Field. Pools of thick, dark energy swirled above her forehead. Slightly behind this spot I perceived an egg-shaped blot. The entire system pulsed, including this blot and the dark energy surrounding it. Although Susan's doctors had found no medical reason to explain her malady, I sensed that there was a physical condition creating a buildup of pressure inside her skull. I performed an Illumination to clear the imprints for this malady and to extract the dark energy swirling around Susan's head.

When I scanned Susan again, I noticed that the object I had sensed earlier was still present. I insisted that she go back to her physician and have an MRI scan to provide a detailed view of the inside of her skull. Susan's doctors were reluctant. There was nothing to justify an MRI, they said. It is an expensive procedure, and if Susan insisted on having it, she would have to pay for it out of her own pocket. She persevered, and with a smile she told her physicians that her shaman had ordered it. When the films came back they showed a growth the size of an egg next to her pituitary gland, in the center of her head, in a cavity that originally had been no larger than the size of a pea. This cyst had been creating a dangerous buildup of pressure in her brain. Two days later her surgeons successfully removed it and found that it was not malignant. After the surgery they explained to Susan that given the size of this cyst, she would have had a very short time left to live. The surgical intervention could not have been more timely.

TRACKING ENERGY

Shamans are master trackers. I remember being in the Amazon rain forest with two shamans with whom I had been traveling for several days. That morning we decided to hike to a nearby river, where pineapples grew on one of the banks. The monkeys knew this spot, and when the pineapples were ripe they came down from the trees for raucous feasts. The jaguars, of course, also knew the spot, and converged at dusk to stalk the monkeys, which are their favorite meal. We were interested in observing the jaguars and knew that if we missed them, at least we could join the monkeys for pineapples. We were following a trail with a thick ground cover of crimson leaves when one of the shamans stopped abruptly. He pointed to the ground and whispered, "Jaguar tracks." I bent down, but all I could see was the thick blanket of moist leaves and scarlet soil. The other shaman silently nodded, then pointed to a tree nearly twenty feet away and exclaimed, "Jaguar fur." We walked up to the tree and found two hairs stuck to a cut in the bark where some great cat had scratched itself. I had seen nothing until the medicine woman pulled the hairs from the tree, which looked exactly like hundreds of other trees in the forest.

We saw no jaguars that day, and the monkeys had already made quick work of the pineapples. But I did receive two great lessons in tracking. I learned that tracking requires the tracker's unconditional attention. When looking for jaguars, you focus on nothing else. In that way two jaguar hairs can stand out like a piece of glass catching the sun in the desert. The second lesson is that tracking happens over space and also across time. We were tracking events that had happened days before; when we began, the prints were nearly four days old. We followed the feline's tracks through the forest, catching a spot of hair here, a footprint on a moist riverbank there, and occasionally a place where she had lain to rest. On the first day we covered three days of the cat's travel as she meandered lazily through the forest. Each track we observed was more recent and better defined than the last. On the second day we came upon the magnificent spotted creature. She was lounging at the edge of a river, preening herself, completely absorbed in licking her forelegs. When she caught our scent she leapt up into the air and disappeared like mist into the jungle.

In a similar manner, a seer learns to track the cause of illness and emotional distress across time. The seer can discover the incident that caused her client's disease or misfortune. The following technique allows you to track a client's wound of origin, the source event that is responsible for a particular malady. This wound can be a recent event, a childhood trauma, or even an experience from a previous lifetime. The seer tracks across time to the original incident when the wounding occurred. My mentor referred to this as finding the wounded "face" of his patient. I learned the practice by tracking for my own wounded "faces."

When I first began to practice this exercise I was sure that the faces I saw were my own subpersonalities, the many selves that live within me. I was not convinced that these faces were ones of my own past incarnations, from one hundred or one thousand years ago. After years of practice, I came to the conclusion that the difference was more a matter of semantics than of reality. There is no hard evidence that we have lived former lives, and this exercise does not constitute proof of previous incarnations. Whether from this or previous life-times, these are the stories that live within me. They are no more or less real to me than the story of my childhood. Whatever their origin, they contain healing power. Such tracking requires a great degree of skill and practice, yet 90 percent of our students achieve this skill by the end of their training.

TRACKING OUR FORMER SELVES

Don Antonio taught me how to use my intent to track. When you are deep in the rain forest following the footprints of jaguars, you exclude everything else from your perceptual horizon. You see dazzling ver-milion and yellow macaw feathers along the way, but you pay them no attention. Your intent is set on jaguars, and everything else blends into the background. Parrot songs and monkey howls are of no con-sequence. Only the growl of the cats interests you. When you are tracking for your own or a client's wound of origin, this is the only face that calls you. Set your intent clearly at the beginning of the tracking session and let Spirit take care of the details. The face that appears still and unchanging after all the earlier transformations is the face that you are tracking for. Once it appears, it will reveal its story to you.

In a darkened room, sit three feet in front of a mirror and place a small candle on a table next to you. Be sure the candle is at your side and not in front of you.

Come into prayer pose, perform the Second Attention eye exer-cise, and become mindful of your breath. When you are completely relaxed, gaze softly into your left eye. Do not stare. Count each inhalation until you reach ten, and then start again at one. Notice the play of light and shadow on your face, and keep focused on your left eye.

There are four stages to the tracking process.

At the first stage notice how your face is as you have always seen it.

Everything is exactly as it appears to be. This is the face you have looked at in the mirror a thousand times.

The second stage begins a few minutes later. Your face may change into different forms. You might perceive animal faces superimposed on yours, or your face may disappear altogether except for your eyes. *Nothing is only what it appears to be in this stage.* Stay with the changes, focusing on your breath. Do not be alarmed by what you perceive. Simply register the various faces that appear, passing no judgment and making no interpretations. Some of them may be tens of thousands of years old. Some may be former lives; others are power animals, our guides and allies in nature. Other faces are our spirit guides.

In the third stage, a single face appears and becomes dominant. *Here everything is as it should be.* This is the face that you are tracking. You have noticed every changing, shape-shifting face until you recognize the face that comes to stillness. When the image appears, allow it to inform you. Hold it steady by focusing on your breath, gazing softly into your left eye. Let it reveal its story to you. Who is it? Where did it come from? What does it want from you? The Luminous Energy Field holds the memories of all of our former selves, including the faces of who we were when we were hurt or wounded. Often these appear as a former lifetime in which you might have experienced great pain and suffering or perhaps died a violent death. More frequently they are the faces of who we once were, or who we might have become, in this lifetime.

In the fourth stage all images disappear, even your own face. At this stage in the tracking practice you are seeing the luminous nature of reality. (I call this the "poof" stage, because everything disappears.) There is only Spirit and light.

To finish the tracking practice, return your hands to prayer pose and take a few deep breaths with your eyes closed.

When I was learning this practice with Don Antonio, he had me work with a fellow student that I disliked greatly. We were a group of twelve that he had selected to train, out of many who had requested to learn from him. Carlos was a man whom I trusted with my life — we had traveled through the mountains and the rain forest together — but I refused to have dinner with him. I found him excessively pious and spiritually trite, and when things did not go his way, he became pouty and infantile. I realized that I was full of judgments about him, but I could not help myself. The dislike was mutual. We avoided each other. Now Antonio had the two of us practicing tracking, looking eye to eye. In the first stage of the process I saw his black eyes and Indian features and was faintly aware of the setting sun and the outline of the mountains behind him. He was in his mid-thirties and had striking black hair, which he had let grow past his shoulders.

In the second stage, his face began to morph. I saw his nose turn into a beak, his eyes recede back into their sockets. In front of my eyes he was changing into a beautiful eagle. Suddenly as I entered the third stage, his face turned into that of a six-year-old. He had tears running down his face and was longing for his mother, who was sick. The little boy seemed bereft, and was convinced his mother would never return home again. He looked inconsolable, and I wanted to reach out and comfort this child.

On the fourth stage I allowed the image to dissolve into pure energy. My partner disappeared, and all I saw were the last rays of the setting sun behind him. Antonio had explained to us that this last stage, which is the most difficult one, was necessary so that we did not bind the enduring image into physical reality. This was particularly important when we were working with a client to track future possibilities. You did not want to lock in the image of a client's destiny. When you dissolved the image, you turned it over to the will of the Great Spirit.

It was difficult to dissolve the image of that forlorn little boy. I could not shake it from my mind. I had to focus on my breathing and let go of the intense feelings this image elicited. At the end of the exercise Carlos and I sat up and hugged each other warmly. We had never done this before. I explained to him the images I had seen, how tender I had felt toward him, and inquired what happened to his mother when he was six. Carlos was a very private man, and since we had avoided each other all these years, we knew nothing of the other's personal life. He explained to me that his mother had died when he was one, while giving birth to his sister. He could not relate at all to what I had seen. At the end of the session Don Antonio explained that what we had seen in each other's face was our own story. To my surprise, when I returned home I queried my mother and discovered that she had been in and out of hospitals for nearly a year when I was six years old.

Before you attempt this exercise with a client, be sure that you have received adequate training in the luminous healing practices. Above all, complete the practices in this chapter for learning to see with the eyes of the heart. For the time being, use the tracking practice to discover all of the facets of your own being. Become familiar with the faces you carry within you. Should one appear on a client, be sure you can recognize it as your own projection. Often other people serve as a mirror for us to get to know those parts of our psyche we keep hidden from ourselves. Carl Jung referred to these disowned parts as the shadow. Remember that when the waters of a lake are absolutely still, the lake reflects the trees, the sky, and everything around it perfectly. At the slightest breeze, with the smallest ripple in the waters, the lake reflects nothing but itself. To see another with clarity and objectivity, one first must master stillness. The slightest breeze of judgment or interpretation from the rational mind will create a ripple that shatters the Second Awareness and returns us to ordinary perception.

TRACKING FUTURE SELVES

This technique can also be used to track into the future, to access a destiny in which you are healed and leading a creative, fulfilling life.

Simply put your intent into tracking possible futures instead of your past. We have many possible destinies available to us. Think of your lifeline as a solid cord of light reaching from the present back into the past, and extending into the future as luminous strands, like fiber-optic threads. Each strand represents a possible future. In one possible future you might live a long and healthy life, but only if you follow through with plans to move to a certain town, accept a certain job or position, or go through a particular change in lifestyle. A different strand might lead you to a less fortunate destiny.

Physicist Werner Heisenberg developed a key principle of quantum mechanics: that one could determine either the velocity or the position of an electron accurately, but not both. The Heisenberg uncertainty principle states that the act of observing an event influences its outcome or destiny. Heisenberg's discovery seems to indicate that the ability to change the physical world through the exercise of vision is very limited once energy has manifested into form. The time to change the world is before form has emerged from the formless, before energy has manifested into matter. Thus many of the healing practices developed by shamans heal conditions before they manifest in the body, before old imprints in the Luminous Energy Field have organized matter into illness or misfortune.

Some seers are able to assist their clients in selecting a destiny that defies their odds for recovery. When working with a client who has a grim health prognosis, I track for alternative futures, among which is a healed state that, although not probable, is permissible within the laws of biology and physics. When I see the healed condition, I can help the odds for recovery become greater. Once that state is identified, the journey toward healing can begin. The story of Steve helps to illustrate this point.

Steve was a physicist working at the Linear Accelerator at Stanford University when he came to see me. He and his colleagues had been analyzing data to determine if enough matter existed in the Universe for it to continue expanding for eternity, or if the gravitational pull of stars was great enough to make the Universe collapse into itself. He took a break from his research to join me in an expedition to the Southwest. We were camping in Canyon de Chelly in Arizona, home today to the Navajo nation. The original canyon dwellers lived in cliff houses above the desert floor until 1200 C.E. When we arrived at the box canyon where we were camping that evening, I cautioned the group to be respectful of the Anasazi burial ground that lay along one wall against a cliff. Over the centuries the rain and the wind had exposed the tombs. In places pottery shards and bone fragments lay along the arid surface. Not even the current occupants of the canyon, the Navajo, ventured near that spot. They believed bad luck befell anyone who disturbs ancient burial sites.

As I was setting up my tent I heard Steve joking with a few of the members of the group, performing the "Alas, poor Yorick" routine from Hamlet. He was holding a human skull in his hands. I ran to him and asked him to return the skull to the site where he had found it. Our Navajo guides were aghast at Steve's antics, and suggested he say a prayer when he took back the skull. They advised that we leave the area as soon as possible.

Two months later I received a call from Steve. "How are things on the research front?" I asked. The news was good. The Universe seemed poised to live forever.

"And how are you?"

For Steve the news was not encouraging. He had been diagnosed a few days earlier with a very advanced case of lymphoma. The doctors at Stanford University Medical Center gave him less than four months to live.

Steve was convinced that the incident with the Anasazi skull was responsible for his cancer. Even though he must have had the cancer for months before the expedition, both of us were moved by the synchronicity of these events. An actual connection between the two events was not important. The significant thing was that Steve *believed* there was a connection between them. Understanding this connection would become part of his healing journey. We began working together immediately after his diagnosis and throughout his chemotherapy. By the end of the fourth month Steve's cancer was in check. Contrary to his prognosis, he was alive. To us this meant that there was a possibility he would live a great deal longer. Granted, it was not very probable, but nevertheless it was possible.

We began to track to find the face of his healed self. We employed the tracking technique, but with an interesting twist. Instead of my tracking for Steve, I merely sat across from him in stillness. Steve had worked with me extensively and was familiar with tracking. I had him use me as a mirror for himself. We knew that he was the one who had to find his healed self. No one can heal you; you heal yourself. All that I could offer Steve were the maps I had learned, but I knew a map was not the territory. He would have to travel the terrain himself. Every time we met we would track. At the end of each session I performed an Illumination, to clear the imprints associated with any of the wounded faces he had discovered. My own stillness served as a tuning fork so that he would not allow himself to be seduced by the beautiful or terrible images he perceived. Most were the faces of his own past—faces of grief, trauma, joy, and loss. He had two young daughters, and he had just met the woman he considered his soul partner; they were to be married the following summer.

Eventually Steve discovered his own stillness. His waters were becoming quiet and beginning to reflect his healed self. Finally, one morning, I saw myself reflected in his eyes, and knew Steve had found what he was looking for. At the end of our practice we simply hugged each other, tears running down our faces. I asked Steve what he had seen, and he replied that he had witnessed everything. I pressed him to explain, and he repeated, "Everything, with a capital E, and myself."

When Steve found his healed self he discovered his original face, his essential nature. I ended up performing the couple's wedding ceremony that summer. Steve lived for another eight years. They were the most important years of his life. A year before he passed away, he sent me a necklace with an orca carved on it, similar to the motifs carved by the Eskimos. The note that arrived with it said that he chose an orca because although they are known as killer whales, they are in fact one of the gentlest of sea animals. They plumb the depths of the ocean, as he had had to plumb the depths of his own soul. They scare the living daylights out of anyone who gets close to them. So too had his cancer, but in reality it had brought him the gift of life.

Very few shamans attain the wisdom and the skill to track someone else's destiny. Only when you know your own essential nature, when you have tracked for your own original face, are you then able to assist another with the absolute nonattachment and compassion this kind of tracking requires. Everything in life leaves its track in time.

CHAPTER 6

SACRED SPACE

INVOCATION

To the winds of the South
Great serpent,
Wrap your coils of light around us,
Teach us to shed the past the way you shed your skin,
To walk softly on the Earth. Teach us the Beauty Way.

To the winds of the West
Mother jaguar,
Protect our medicine space.
Teach us the way of peace, to live impeccably
Show us the way beyond death.

To the winds of the North.
Hummingbird, Grandmothers and Grandfathers,
Ancient Ones
Come and warm your hands by our fires
Whisper to us in the wind
We honor you who have come before us,
And you who will come after us, our children's children.

To the winds of the East.
Great eagle, condor
Come to us from the place of the rising Sun.

Keep us under your wing.
Show us the mountains we only dare to dream of.
Teach us to fly wing to wing with the Great Spirit.

Mother Earth.
We've gathered for the healing of all of your children.
The Stone People, the Plant People.
The four-legged, the two-legged, the creepy crawlers.
The finned, the furred, and the winged ones.
All our relations.

Father Sun, Grandmother Moon, to the Star Nations.
Great Spirit, you who are known by a thousand names
And you who are the unnamable One.
Thank you for bringing us together
And allowing us to sing the Song of Life.

PRAYER FOR CREATING SACRED SPACE

SHAMANS ALWAYS BEGIN HEALING CEREMONIES BY OPENING SACRED space. In this space we leave behind the affairs of ordinary life, the bustling world of meetings and schedules, and prepare to meet the divine. Sacred space allows us to enter our quiet inner world where healing takes place. Here the mundane cannot distract us, and every act is hallowed and deliberate; yet sacred space is neither serious nor ponderous. Shamans take their work very seriously, but they do not take themselves very seriously at all, and there is often laughter and playfulness during healing ceremonies. Within sacred space we experience the lightness of our being. Both laughter and tears come easily. Alan Watts used to say that the reason angels could fly was because they took themselves very lightly. Within sacred space our burdens become lighter, and we can be touched by the hand of

Spirit. After we finish our healing work, sacred space must be closed by again acknowledging the four directions, Heaven, and Earth. When the shaman does this, she releases the archetypal energies she summoned, and they reintegrate into nature.

Sacred space is a healing sphere that is pure, holy, and safe. I imagine it as a shimmering cupola above the area where I do my healing work. Everyone within this space is protected, and my client can release grief and pain and experience the joy that often accompanies the healing process. Much of our fear and pain derives from the feeling that the world is not a safe place for us. When the world is dangerous and predatory we raise our defenses. Our psychological armor goes on. Sacred space creates an environment where our defenses can be lowered, where we can explore our soft, tender underbelly. Sacred space also gives us access to the luminous healers—the medicine men and women who assist us from the Spirit world.

We are taught early on that the sacred is found inside temples, cathedrals, or perhaps a beautiful spot in nature. Do the four walls of a church create sacred space? Is it the prayers that have been uttered there over the years? How many prayers does it take to make a space sacred? Perhaps one prayer spoken from the heart is enough. You can create sacred space and summon the healing power of nature anywhere on Earth. I use the invocation at the beginning of this chapter. I did not learn it from anyone, although it has elements in it, such as the four directions and their archetypal animals, that are shared by many Native American peoples. It is novel and ancient at the same time. You can use it while your own prayer reveals itself to you. Although there are certain components necessary to create sacred space, you can in time bring in your own personal expression. For example, notice that the prayer is anchored in the spatial directions. It calls on the four points of the compass, and above and below. The six directions plus the shaman in the center represent the seven organizing principles of the Universe. Serpent represents the binding principle; jaguar is the renewing force; hummingbird represents the epic journey of evolution and growth; and eagle or condor stands for the self-transcending principle. Heaven is the creative force; Earth is the receptive force. When you summon them, you align yourself with the forces that animate all life.

The shaman's covenant with Spirit is that when she calls, Spirit answers. Powerful medicine people from the Spirit world appear in the form of luminous beings who assist us in our healing work. Literally we use the four cardinal directions to get our bearings in the material world. We travel north to see polar bears, go south for the winter, move to the East or West Coast. For the shaman, these directions also personalize qualities and energies. If we can imagine the movement of these energies in the same way that the evening weather forecast shows the jet stream bringing rain from one area to another, we can understand how energy moves through space. The qualities of each of the four directions are represented by archetypal animals. These creatures are more than symbols; they are primordial energies or spirits. Each archetype has a life and powers of its own. The archetypal animals of the cardinal directions vary among Native cultures in the Americas. For me the hummingbird represents the North direction, whereas for certain North American indigenous peoples it is buffalo. While the representations vary from culture to culture, the properties of these energies remains the same because they stand for the same organizing principles of nature. The important thing is not what we call these energies, or even which archetype we use, but that we get to know them well enough that when we call, they respond. The call comes from the heart; the voice is our love, Spirit responds. When we call within sacred space, the Universe conspires on our behalf.

I met Father Alexander, a priest from Chicago, when he enrolled in our training program. Two years after I met him he was called by his bishop to take charge of a church where the rector had become ill. The church had undertaken a major restoration project. The roof was leaking, and the stained-glass windows needed an overhaul. Unfortunately, the parish had run out of funds. To complicate matters, the congregation had been shrinking; a lack of parking space made it difficult for elderly parishioners to walk to church when snow and ice covered the ground.

A few days after he arrived at his post, when no one was in the church, Father Alexander opened sacred space above the main altar, calling in the four directions, the Heavens, and Mother Earth. Feeling that he was in an untenable situation, like a captain assigned to a sinking ship, he was willing to try anything. He determined to leave the space open for a month to see if this would bring any change. The following week, as he and a fellow priest explored the various rooms in the complex, they came to a door that would not budge. They called a carpenter, who had to remove the door from the frame. They discovered that the closed passageway led to the belfry, a room half the size of a basketball court, which to their dismay lay buried six feet deep in bat excrement. In addition to the health hazard, the sheer weight of the droppings threatened to collapse the belfry. Things seemed to be going from bad to worse.

Father Alexander went to the main altar, reopened the sacred space, and called in an expert to dispose of the decades-long accumulation of bat droppings. After examining the mountain of guano, the man informed Father Alexander that $40,000 was the best price he could offer. The priest shook his head in dismay. The expert looked confused, then explained that he was willing to pay $40,000 for the guano. It seems that bat droppings make the best fertilizer but are extremely hard to come by in any quantity. Father Alexander was elated. They were able to repair the roof before winter arrived. Days later, they convinced the city to permit Sunday parking in the police department's lot across the street. As a result, Father Alexander has become in great demand in the Archdiocese of Chicago. Periodically he is called to help other churches in distress. Whenever he goes to a new church he opens sacred space at the main altar. He is convinced that when he does so, Spirit accepts his invitation to lend him a much-needed hand. Within sacred space we have extraordinary spiritual assistance available to us.

THE POWER ANIMALS

SERPENT

Each of the archetypal animals exudes a different flavor of energy. In the South serpent symbolizes knowledge, sexuality, and healing. Perhaps the most universal archetype, serpent has always represented the healing power of nature. The staff of medicine, or caduceus, is formed by two serpents intertwined around a rod. Moses carried a serpent staff when he led the Israelites through the desert. In Western mythology a serpent brought us the fruit of the tree of knowledge. In the East it is the coiled snake of the Kundalini energy.

Serpent represents the primeval connection to the feminine and thus is a symbol of fertility and sexuality. Serpent does not represent sex per se; this is a common misconception. Rather it symbolizes the essential life force that seeks union and creation. Remember that every cell in our body seeks to divide and procreate. In nature, fecundity is the creative principle of the cosmos. We can summon the creative principle from the South by calling on the archetype of serpent. When I work with a client who has lost her passion for life, who has exhausted her energy and enthusiasm, I connect her with the energies of the South and send her home accompanied by the spirit of serpent. I know that this will rekindle her longing for life.

JAGUAR

The animal of the West is jaguar. It renews and transforms the life of the rain forest. Whereas serpent represents the power of healing, which is gradual and incremental, jaguar stands for sudden transformation, life and death. It might seem odd to us that the transforming force in the Universe is also associated with death, yet to the ancient Americans these two energies were cut from the same cloth. That which endured was always changing and renewing itself. That which remained unchanging perished. They knew that stable, steady states were only temporary, because everything in the Universe is in flux. In North America, shamans set fire to the underbrush, unleashing in a controlled manner the forces represented by jaguar. This prevented lightning from starting a fire that would consume the entire forest. They recognized that chaos and order, expansion and contraction, were the natural cycle of life.

When we get sick we have an opportunity not only to regain our health but to make a quantum leap to an even greater level of wellness. Healing is a method not only for eliminating symptoms but for achieving increasingly higher states of health. I have worked with clients in their sixties and seventies who tell me that they have never felt better in their lives. This is the energy of jaguar. A stable system does not change easily. People generally change not when things are going right but when things are going wrong. Crisis, therefore, becomes a time of opportunity. We can transform our bodies so that they heal more rapidly and age more elegantly by embodying the forces represented by jaguar. I have grown to believe in the metaphor that we have nine lives, like cats. When we reach the end of one of these lifetimes (other people would call them stages or phases in one's life), it's important to give the old self a decent burial, and then leap like a jaguar into who we are becoming. Otherwise, we can spend years patching and fixing an old self that we have outgrown.

The jungle cat is the steward of the rain forest and keeper of the gateway of death. Jaguar helps to dismember that which must die in order for the new to be born. A hurricane embodies the chaotic power of jaguar. A beehive or ant colony with its complexity and beauty displays the organizing power of jaguar. Jaguar energy works at the level of a village, an organization, or an individual. Sometimes a marriage needs to be dissolved in order for the parties to survive and be healthy. Sometimes a village must be abandoned so that its members can thrive in a different location. All through the Americas we find archeological evidence of villages being deserted for no reason apparent to us. They did this in response to the cyclical nature of order and chaos. The Anasazi in the American Southwest, the Maya, and the Inka periodically abandoned their homes to build new villages elsewhere.

A few years ago, when a wildfire burned out of control through the highland jungle around Machu Picchu, firefighters battled the flames for days. The flames leapt uncontrollably from one ridge to the other and consumed tens of thousands of acres. This was the dry season, when it never rains in this part of the Andes. When the fire was within a few hundred yards of Machu Picchu, a medicine woman arrived to perform a ceremony at the ruins. Everyone took part in the ritual, even the archeologists. As the fire entered the Inka City of Light, the sky suddenly grew overcast and the rains came and extinguished the fire. The shaman claimed it was the spirit of the rain forest herself, in the form of a jaguar, that responded to her call and brought the rains. I believe her ceremony brought balance to the land, and the rains came.

There is a legend from Bali of a village where it had not rained for six years. None of their shamans was able to bring the rains back — they were too enmeshed in the local patterns and so could not influence it. Fields were scorched, and the villagers were tired of living off the generosity of their neighbors. A shaman from a village two mountains away was summoned to assist. When she arrived she noticed the misery around her. She asked the villagers for a hut where she could fast and meditate. On the third day, as she came out of her hut, the sky had grown dark with clouds, and thunderclaps echoed through the valley. A few moments later the rains came. The entire village came out to celebrate. Everyone was dancing in the rain. When the elders inquired what she had done, she replied: "When I arrived, your village was so out of balance that I became out of balance. This is why I had to go into the hut to fast and pray. When I came back into balance, your village returned to balance and the rains came."

When I work with a client in crisis, who may feel his life is beyond repair, I send him home with jaguar. Often my client thinks this is only a metaphor. I know that the life-and-death principle represented by the jaguar will assist him to allow those parts of himself that need to die to do so, as well as to regain hope and bring new balance from chaos. Jaguar energy can be summoned to contain the chaotic spread of a cancer or of a fire through the forest. It can be summoned to assist a dying person find peace in the chaos that accompanies the dying process, and guide her journey back to the world of Spirit.

Jungle people also revere jaguar because it can transform heavy energies within the Luminous Energy Field. Legends say that when jaguar enters a ceremony, it devours the negative emotions of anger, fear, and grief. Jaguar is a spiritual cleanup crew, transforming thick, heavy energies into light. As the protector of all life, jaguar safeguards the ceremonial space against any negative energies that could penetrate your healing circle. When a client needs spiritual or psychological protection, I connect him with jaguar energy. Often he reports seeing a large medicine cat in his dreams. To use this energy to heal or bring balance to life we must become personally acquainted with the spirit of jaguar.

Hummingbird

In the North direction, hummingbird represents the courage required to embark on an epic journey. Hummingbirds migrate over the Atlantic, traveling every year from Brazil to Canada. At first glance, the hummingbird would not seem suited for transatlantic flight. It does not have eagle's majestic wingspan, nor can its little body store much in the way of food. Yet it responds to an ancestral call to embark on this epic flight. It responds to the call each year in the same way that salmon return upstream to the site where they were spawned. When I work with a client who is embarking upon an epic life journey, I help her to connect with the energy of hummingbird. This is not only an inspiring metaphor for a journey but an energetic connection with this nature principle. Once touched by the energies of this archetype, we are propelled on our own epic journey that eventually leads us back to our source, where our spirit was spawned. In that ancestral field of flowers, we can drink deeply from the nectar of our lives.

The North energy helps us embark on great journeys despite tremendous odds. When there is not enough time, money, or know-how for what you are attempting, hummingbird can provide the courage and guidance necessary for success.

Archeologists know that the first Americans crossed the land bridge over the Bering Strait thousands of years ago. They traversed Alaska, then descended into what is now Canada and the United States. What propelled the early Americans to cross a frigid ice shelf to come into the New World? Why, after this great crossing, did they not remain in North America, where they found lush forests and abundant game, but set off instead on an arduous journey across the barren deserts of northern Mexico to populate the rest of the American continents? Living beings seek to explore and discover. This instinct is operant in every one of us. When we deny the call of hummingbird, we begin to die. When we settle for comfort over discovery, or compromise the soul's longing to grow, we begin to wither. When we reawaken the great instinct to learn and explore, our lives grow less trivial and mundane and become epic.

EAGLE

The East direction is represented by eagle and condor, who bring vision, clarity, and foresight. Eagle perceives the entire panorama of life without becoming bogged down in its details. The energies of eagle assist us in finding the guiding vision of our lives. The eyes of condor see into the past and the future, helping to know where we come from, and who we are becoming. When I work with a client who is stuck in the traumas of the past, I help her to connect with the spirit of eagle or condor. As this energy infuses the healing space, my client is often able to attain new clarity and insight into her life. This is not an intellectual insight, but rather a call, faint at first, hardly consciously heard. Her possibilities beckon to her and propel her out of her grief and into her destiny.

I believe that while everyone has a future, only certain people have a destiny. Having a destiny means living to your fullest human potential. You don't need to become a famous politician or poet, but your destiny has to be endowed with meaning and purpose. You could be a street sweeper and be living a destiny. You could be the president of a large corporation and be living a life bereft of meaning. One can make oneself available to destiny, but it requires a great deal of courage to do so. Otherwise our destiny bypasses us, leaving us deprived of a fulfillment known by those who choose to take the road less traveled. Eagle allows us to rise above the mundane battles that occupy our lives and consume our energy and attention. Eagle gives us wings to soar above trivial day-to-day struggles into the high peaks close to Heaven. Eagle and condor represent the self-transcending principle in nature.

Biologists have identified the self-transcending principle as one of the prime agendas of evolution. Living molecules seek to transcend their selfhood to become cells, then simple organisms, which then form tissues, then organs, and then evolve into complex beings such as humans and whales. Every transcending jump is inclusive of all of the levels beneath it. Cells are inclusive of molecules, yet transcend them; organs are inclusive of cells, yet go far beyond them; whales are inclusive of organs yet cannot be described by them, as the whole transcends the sum of its parts.

The transcending principle represented by eagle states that problems at a certain level are best solved by going up one step. The problems of cells are best resolved by organs, while the needs of organs are best addressed by an organism such as a butterfly or a human. The same principle operates in our lives. Think of nested Russian dolls. Material needs are the tiny doll in the center. The larger emotional doll encompasses them, and both are contained within the outermost spiritual doll. In this way, we cannot satisfy emotional needs with material things, but we can satisfy them spiritually. When we go one step up, our emotional needs are addressed in the solution. We rise above our life dilemmas on the wings of eagle and see our lives in perspective.

HEAVEN AND EARTH

The final two directions, above and below, represent the masculine and feminine. The Sun in the sky is the creative life force. Ancient peoples observed that while the sky appeared to move in the course of the night and the seasons, the stars themselves were unchanging. The constellations were always in the same relationship with each other. The sun rose in the east in the same location on every summer solstice. In the Inka traditions all prayers are addressed first to the South direction, as the Southern Cross is the one point in the sky that remains unchanging as all the other stars rotate during the night. (The North Star is not visible from the Southern Hemisphere, so all orientations are toward the south.) The power of Heaven is the unchanging. The shaman summons it to preserve and perpetuate, while understanding that life is a delicate balance between the changing and the unchanging. The Inka believe that the soul has three parts. When people die, one part of their soul (the changing) returns to the Earth to be reabsorbed into nature and become one with all life. Another part (their power and wisdom) returns to the sacred mountains, and a third part (the unchanging) returns to the

Sun. Many of the shaman's advanced rites of passage are meant to help one recognize that part of themselves that returns to the Sun and is perpetual and unchanging.

Earth is the receptive and nurturing principle. Its power is to mulch and renew. The summer leaves are turned back into rich soil. The bodies of the ancestors are absorbed back into the ecosphere and become one with the trees, the pastures, and the mountains. Seeds germinate within the dark, fertile folds of Mother Earth. All life emerges from her moist womb and is nurtured by her abundance. The changing seasons represent the mutable quality of Earth. In the story of Genesis, the Earth and the Heavens were one in the beginning. Thus the changing contains the unchanging within it. The dark womb of space contains the sun. Even though the leaves of springtime were mulched back into the Earth in the fall, it was to bring about the new life after the winter. Summoning the energies of Heaven and Earth reconnects us with the natural cycles of our lives. But most important, it allows us to embrace the mother who will always nurture us and the father who will never leave us. Coming home to the primeval mother and father is tremendously healing of childhood wounds. Many of my clients who have issues of abandonment undergo enormous change simply by embracing Mother Earth and Father Sky as their natural parents. I always assist my clients to connect with the energies of Heaven and Earth, regardless of the condition or issue for which they came to see me. When saluting the Earth we acknowledge our relationship with all other life forms, from the trees to the fishes, the birds, and the stones. When saluting the Heavens we acknowledge our star brothers and sisters, and we dedicate our healing effort to the Great Spirit, the Creator of all.

OPENING SACRED SPACE

Use the invocation at the beginning of the chapter. You can employ a smudge stick of sage or a little scented water if you like. Shamans throughout the Americas accompany their prayers by fanning smoldering sage or incense with a feather in the appropriate direction, blowing a few drops of scented water toward the direction they are addressing, or holding their hand up to the sky and saluting each cardinal point. You will need to determine the points; ideally this is done with a compass, but a close approximation based on your knowledge of the landscape is fine.

Begin by facing South. Smudge or blow the scented water to the South, then hold up your hand, palm facing out. Recite the first verse, calling upon serpent. Face each direction in turn as you repeat the process. Touch the Earth and look to the Heavens when directing your prayers there. You close sacred space by thanking serpent, jaguar, hummingbird, and eagle. Release their energies and allow them to return to the four corners of the Earth. To connect with the energy of one of the directions, do not close that direction. Instead, call on that archetype to enter you and accompany you on your path. (I do this by turning to the East, for example, and instead of closing that direction I blow the spirit of that archetype into my client's crown chakra. I imagine the spirit of eagle entering them and informing their lives.) Then thank Mother Earth and Father Sky.

EXPANDING YOUR LUMINOUS ENERGY FIELD

Besides calling in the directions, there is another powerful way that we can create sacred space. We do this is by utilizing the light of the eighth chakra, above the head. The power of sacred space is amplified many times when we expand this radiant orb and rest within it. The eighth chakra resides inside the Luminous Energy Field, outside the physical body. It is that part of us that is always one with God. When we expand it like a crystal dome, we can actually sit within it and shield ourselves from the static of the world.

Imagine your eighth chakra like a small radiant sun above your head. Some people experience either a hot or cool sensation when they feel its membrane. Note its pulse and frequency. Does it seem to vibrate? Does it have a rhythm? Use your imagination to picture an orb the color of the rising sun. Imagine its brilliance shimmering on the surface, rippling across it like waves, bathing you in orange and yellows.

Bring your hands over your chest into prayer pose. Slowly raise your hands, still in prayer pose, until they are above your head. Sense your fingertips entering the globe of the eighth chakra. Sense how this spinning sun yields and opens to you. Very slowly, like a peacock opening its fan, expand the circumference of this brilliant orb to envelop you by turning your palms outward and extending your arms. Bring your arms down until your hands touch the chair, and bask in the light of your eighth chakra.

Experience yourself within this luminous sphere. Sense the quiet and stillness that pervades this space. Pay attention to your breathing. Follow your inhalation and then exhale softly. Explore the inside of this radiant orb with your awareness. What does the inner membrane feel like? I imagine it like a great bubble, with tides of color washing through it, yet with a distinct radiance of its own, like a sun. This is the vessel that houses your soul in between incarnations. When you have explored this space to your satisfaction, with arms outstretched bring your hands up slowly, like a peacock closing its fan, until you have gathered this luminous chakra again above your head. Feel it glowing. Bring your hands again over your chest to prayer pose to conclude the exercise.

It is important always to close sacred space after you have completed your work. Gather the luminous orb of your eighth chakra to its place above your head. Release the spirits of serpent, jaguar, hummingbird, and eagle. Thank Heaven and Earth. When we do not close sacred space we contaminate it, like polluting a freshwater spring. The archetypal animals no longer come to you, and the forces of nature stop responding to your call.

Invoke sacred space with the greatest respect. Holding sacred space is like holding the tone of a single note. Your song must be true and crystalline for its quality to be pure. When you are in the presence of a master shaman or a great spiritual teacher, you feel a difference in the quality of the space. The energy is clean; there is a magnetism in the room. It requires all of our love and intent, as well as practice, to hold sacred space for more than a few moments. With practice, though, it becomes effortless. The space sustains itself.

PART III

THE

SHAMAN'S

WORK

Before you attempt the following techniques with a client, be sure that you have received adequate training in the luminous healing practices. The Illumination and Extraction Processes require a degree of mastery one acquires only from supervised practice. The Illumination Process metabolizes the heavy energies that congest a chakra. It burns up toxic residues and clears the imprints of disease in the Luminous Energy Field. I insist that my students master the art of holding sacred space before they practice an Illumination. This is the equivalent of a sterile field where you perform surgery. No amount of surgical technique will help if you have a contaminated field. Infection will set in, and your patient can become critically ill. Similarly, sacred space creates a safe environment where noxious energies cannot penetrate. I let my students know that when their sacred space collapses, they can endanger themselves and their clients. You maintain sacred space through the focus of intent. This is why having a meditation or yoga practice is so helpful. Meditators have learned to still their mind and focus their awareness. In a study done several years ago, Zen meditators were able to maintain the alpha state (with their brain waves at around eight cycles per second) uninterruptedly. When a loud noise shattered the calm, their meditative state was broken, but within seconds they were able to reenter the alpha state. On the other hand, when nonmeditators were distracted by a loud noise, they were unable to recover their calm until minutes later, if at all.

The Extraction Process allows you to remove energies that have crystallized and become embedded in your client's body. This technique requires a finely developed kinesthetic sense. It also helps if the healer has developed the Second Awareness, the shaman's way of seeing. The process extracts intrusive energies or entities that may be afflicting your client. I find that many people have an aversion to the thought of intrusive energies and entities. We prefer to think of the invisible world as populated only by beneficent luminous beings. I encourage my students to not allow their preconceptions to interfere with their experience. It may be shocking to realize that there are disturbing energies and entities that can affect us, but it is a great relief to know that there are ways that we can help heal those that are suffering from these conditions. I have found that the Extraction Process can accomplish in one session what often could not be achieved in years of psychotherapy.

You do not have to be a shaman to perform the Death Rites. It is my heartfelt wish that you never have to practice these rites. The truth is that most of us will have to assist a loved one in his or her journey to the world of Spirit. Study these rites now so that you develop a feel for them. Assisting a parent in his or her final crossing is the greatest gift that you can give to the person who brought you into this world.

CHAPTER 7

THE ILLUMINATION PROCESS

Three days into the fast. Found the cave almost by accident, after searching the undergrowth for hours. It had started to rain, when I saw an overhang of rock that I thought would provide shelter. Antonio had sent me to find the Temple of the Moon, on the backside of Machu Picchu. "Careful with the vipers," he said as he waved goodbye, a smile on his lips. I sometimes don't understand his sense of humor. Have not seen a single snake, although I am cut and bruised from scrambling through the undergrowth. No trails here. Only the faint remains of a granite step here or a collapsed terrace there.

The cavern is the size of a school bus, with stunning Inka stonework. Dozens of niches carved into the wall. In the back, where two of the walls intersect in an angle, the stone masons cut increasingly smaller triangular stones that fit together perfectly without mortar. The smallest one at the top is no bigger than a matchbox. The entire place is overgrown with moss, but it's dry.

Antonio had commented that I am a weeder and that he was a gardener. He charged me with always working on healing my faults, digging my hurt up like weeds. Nothing beautiful grew in the garden of my soul, he said. I did not know how to water the seeds of my spirit, of who I could become. So he sent me to this cave on a vision quest, to fast for five days. The last two days I've spent weeding the cave. Turns out I do that pretty well. The ground is clear now, rich, dark soil that compacts easily.

Threw away the Hershey bar at the bottom of my pack this

morning. Unwrapped, it, pocketed the foil, and tossed the choco-
late into the jungle. All I had been thinking of for the last two
days was that piece of chocolate.

Antonio is right, I am a weeder, and my life is a jungle, tan-
gled and overgrown. Stuff just grows in it. Sometimes exotic
plants, most of the time vines and creepers that I get tangled in.
Takes all my energy to keep the ground beneath me cleared. How
do I plant the fruit trees and flowers I want to grow old with?

JOURNALS

WESTERN MYTHOLOGY TELLS US THAT WE LIVE IN A PREDATORY UNI-
verse where we are constantly being stalked by "bad" microbes and
hungry jaguars. Medicine people, on the other hand, believe that we
live in a benign universe. The world becomes predatory only when
we are out of balance. The world today is out of balance. Our people
and our crops are besieged by predatory microbes and viruses. Our
antibiotic arsenals are quickly proving ineffective. The Illumination
Process brings us back into balance, into what Inka shamans call
ayni, or proper relationship, with jaguars, microbes, and all life, so
that the Universe again can work on our behalf.

The Illumination Process achieves healing in three ways. First, it
burns up the sludge and deposits adhering to the walls of a chakra.
This promotes longevity and strengthens the immune response. Second, it combusts the toxic energy around malignant physical and
emotional imprints. This is the fuel that an imprint employs to
express itself. Third, it scours clean the imprints in the Luminous
Energy Field. The Illumination Process brings about healing at the
source, at the blueprint level of our being. When these imprints are
erased, one can readily change negative emotions and behaviors. The
power of the immune system is unleashed, so that physical healing is
accelerated.

Every imprint in the Luminous Energy Field is linked to a chakra through which it releases its toxic data into the central nervous system. The imprint is the source, the chakra the pipeline, and the nervous system the distribution network. Each chakra contains a map of the emotional and physical landscape of our life. In the same way that a mountain range can be described in a number of ways—by an aerial map, or by a contour map showing the different strata of the land, or by a population density map—the chakras contain maps of our life experience interpreted through their various lenses. In the first chakra are the survival maps. In the second chakra are the emotional maps, and so forth. To better understand a client's problem, I perform a chakra assessment to determine which is the compromised energy center. This tells me through which chakra an imprint in the Luminous Energy Field informs the emotional and physical well-being of my client.

COMBUSTING ENERGIES

Buckminster Fuller used to say that as the Earth circles the Sun, bands of sunlight wrap around the branches and trunks of trees. He explained that when we ignite a log in our fireplace we are setting that sunlight free again. Everything living is light bound into matter. Whales eat plankton that feeds on light. We eat plants that feast on light. The animals we consume eat plants that feed on light. Everything is made of light, even the dark energies that clog chakras and fuel imprints. Like a log that must be put in the fire for its light to be released, these energies need to be combusted (or extracted, as we will learn in the next chapter). Shamans in the Andes refer to this process as *mihuy*, which means "to digest" or "to combust."

In the Inka shamanic traditions there are no "bad" energies. There are only energies that are "light," and so support life, and energies that are "heavy," which cannot be digested. Your Luminous Energy Field will combust energies naturally and automatically when you envelop a client within it. The residues that cannot be combusted are returned to the Earth, like the ashes from a fire. The Illumination Process unbinds the light trapped within matter. There is no danger of picking up or absorbing any negativity from the client if you are working within sacred space. Legends say that the spirit of jaguar assists you in mulching these energies back into light. The light released from combustion, from *mihuy*, is reabsorbed by your client and replenishes the fuel reserves in his or her Luminous Energy Field.

The Illumination Process transforms heavy energies into light. This is also a metaphor for saying that it transforms emotional wounds into sources of power and knowledge. In mythology, this is the way of the wounded healer. Through an alchemical process (*mihuy*) one transforms one's wounds into a source of courage and strength. I know that every emotional wound with which a client comes to me contains valuable lessons. Once these lessons are learned, the client no longer needs to relive the painful experience. The wounds cease scripting reality and turn out to be gifts of love and strength. What was once a crippling story can be transformed into newfound peace and compassion. The healer can empathize with another's pain because she knows what it is like to hurt. No longer crippled by the past, she is inspired by it, no matter how difficult or painful. When integrated, these experiences temper the steel of one's soul.

I met Gail, a Jungian psychologist from Houston, when she signed up for our healing training program. I was immediately impressed by her generosity and compassion. She always made time for anyone in need, and she had a smile and a kind word for all. I had no idea that she had lost her twenty-four-year-old daughter to a sudden illness a few years earlier. After her tragic loss, Gail hardly left her house. She lost her desire to live, and what little food she took in she ate alone in her room. There was nothing her husband could do to help her out of her despair. Gail would spend many hours every day in contemplation. One year after her daughter's passing, Gail came out of her gloom. Her depression had lifted. That year in solitude had brought her the realization that her destiny was to help as many people in need as she could. Since then she has become a leading advocate of the Dalai Lama in America. She has personally assisted countless Tibetans to relocate in the United States.

During her year of mourning Gail discovered the courage to make a difference in the world. She has touched the lives of countless people across the world. But above all, she is a model of a woman who faced loss and grief and came out stronger on the other side. She not only integrated the lessons that life brought her. She managed to turn a personal tragedy into a source of strength and compassion.

The lessons are integrated at an energetic level. When toxic energies in a chakra are combusted, the natural seeds of that chakra can grow. When fear no longer lives in our belly, compassion blossoms; when scarcity no longer resides in our first chakra, we experience the abundant love of the Universe. When grief no longer dwells in our third chakra, we can change the world. Our luminous architecture changes. Weeks later intellectual understanding follows. In our work, understanding always follows healing. Change happens first at a core energetic level, and then the intellect gets it. In contrast, in the West we insist that understanding must precede healing. We first rehash and rationalize how our mother or father was not emotionally available for us before we embark on change. In luminous healing, the mind can have its insight after the energy field and the body change, but true transformation can never be preceded by the intellect.

The Illumination Process transforms the heavy emotions associated with trauma and disease into nourishing life energy. The by-products of burning wood, for example, are heat and light. Heavy energies are compacted into tight bundles that make them unavailable for use as fuel and life force. Just as we cannot warm ourselves by a log until it is set afire, we cannot clear these dense energies until the Illumination Process unbinds the light within them.

The first step is to burn up the sludge and energetic residues encrusted in the chakra. We must clean out these energies in a chakra in the same way that we would cleanse a cut. When we cut ourselves, we wash the area thoroughly, because if we let dirt accumulate in it, it will become infected and not heal. The same process happens in the Luminous Energy Field. The only difference is that we clean a cut with soap and water, while we cleanse these dark energies with fire. The Illumination Process combusts the energies trapped around an imprint and turns them into light. These energies are the dirt and grime we burn out during the Illumination Process. Once it is clear, the chakra becomes a looking glass into the Luminous Energy Field, and we can read its maps in clear detail. When I employ the Second Awareness I can discern the event that caused the original wounding.

Psychological healing helps to release the emotional energy trapped in an imprint, allowing us to understand the painful incident that caused it. But intellectual understanding does not clear the underlying imprint itself. It is as if a cut were cleaned but never bandaged. Within weeks or months, emotional energy again collects around the imprint and reactivates it. Psychological issues we thought we had healed long ago again rear their ugly heads, and destructive behaviors resurface. (This is a possible explanation for why some people feel the need to continue talk therapy for years; they need to keep cleaning out the wound. And, in fact, recently there has been a surge of interest in the shamanic healing process among psychologists.) After the Illumination Process combusts the energies around the imprint, the underlying imprints are erased. There is no pattern left in the blueprint to reorganize an old reality.

Transforming toxic emotional energies into light is an essential benefit of the Illumination Process, but it is not the entire remedy. After the sludge in the chakra and around the imprint has been combusted, we use clear light to overwrite the information contained in the imprint. This is why I call it the Illumination Process, because when we illuminate the chakra we overwrite the imprint with pure light. We overwrite the imprint with energy from the radiant sun of the eighth chakra. You shower your client's open chakra with a stream of golden sunlight. During this phase a client will often report sensations of peace and deep communion with Spirit. This is the taste of infinity.

The Illumination Process can elicit painful memories. Remember that this is not a psychological process in which a client recalls traumas from the past and speaks about them with a therapist. Illumination is an energetic process. Rather than recounting incidents, the client feels his pain or grief as a wave of energy washing through him. At the end of the healing session, the client is left in a peaceful and often blissful state. I ask my client to recall the emotional intensity of the trauma he is coming to heal. He feels the intensity of the energy but does not relive the emotional pain of the experience and often will not even tell me the full details until after the healing session. If I am working with a client who felt neglected as a child, I ask him to recall the feelings of abandonment or the pain he experienced during the incident. This allows me to follow the luminous tracks left by this event, find the affected chakra, and locate the source of the imprint in the Luminous Energy Field.

I instruct my clients that they are always in control of the process. At times they may feel intense emotions, their hands or legs may cramp, or their bodies might twitch or move involuntarily. If at any time this feels uncomfortable, they can slow the process down by crossing their arms over their chest, right over left. (This is a technique found in every culture for interrupting energy flow. The pharaohs in Egypt were buried in this position to protect them in their journeys to the afterlife, and even today martial artists use it to block a blow.) This lets my clients know that they can regulate the intensity of the experience, and it gives them permission to go as deep as they wish, or to slow down or stop the process altogether.

THE ILLUMINATION PROCESS, STEP BY STEP

The entire process takes about one hour to complete. Only one healing issue and one chakra should be worked on during an Illumination session. These are the steps:

1. Client assessment.
2. Track for imprints.
3. Open sacred space, calling in the directions.
4. Envelop your client in your Luminous Energy Field.
5. Apply deepening points for ten minutes.
6. Open the compromised chakra.
7. Apply release points for five minutes.
8. Extract dense energies from the chakra, flicking to the Earth.
9. Call on jaguar to assist in metabolizing heavy energies.
10. Illuminate to clear the imprint.
11. Balance the chakra and close the Luminous Energy Field.
12. Process with the client.
13. Close the directions.

CLIENT ASSESSMENT

I begin every session by asking my client why she has come to see me. It helps me to identify the energetic issue if I first hear her story. I listen carefully, and we take however long is necessary for my client to feel she has been heard. Oftentimes I will dedicate the entire first hour to this step, but I will not allow it to turn into a psychotherapy session. I am interested in her story but not in analyzing the story. I observe my client's body language carefully, noting where her hands move as she describes her pain or problem, seeking subconscious clues as to the location wherein this imprint resides and the chakra associated with it.

TRACK FOR IMPRINTS

We train our students in the Healing the Light Body School to track imprints in the Luminous Energy Field using applied kinesiology, also known as muscle testing. This technique was developed by Dr. John Diamond, even though versions of muscle testing are also employed by shamans. This procedure is commonly used by chiropractors and other body workers to test skeletal and muscle alignment; I've adapted it for tracking imprints in the Luminous Energy Field. Until you develop your ability to see the inky fields associated with the imprints of disease, this technique is the most practical and reliable I have found. When performed with precision, it accurately reads the condition of a client's energy systems. Since it is the client's body that responds, not the rational mind, you can be relatively certain that you are getting accurate information.

Both healer and client should remove metallic objects — jewelry, watches, and the like. The client closes her eyes and extends one arm horizontally in front of her, so that it is parallel to the ground. Press down with two fingers on the client's wrist while telling her to resist. Most people are able to resist the pressure and maintain their arm extended and parallel to the ground. Next, ask the client to recall someone she loves, and again test her strength. The arm should test strong, as the people we love elicit a dynamic, strengthening response from our energy fields. Then ask the client to recall someone who provokes dislike or fear. The arm should test weak — that is, when you exert pressure with your two fingers the arm should come down toward the ground, as fear and judgment tend to debilitate us. To verify the accuracy of the muscle response, have the client visualize the Dalai Lama, the Buddha, Christ, the Goddess, or whoever most symbolizes love and compassion for her. Again, the muscles should test strong. Visualizing a swastika, which we have learned to associate with the Nazi death camps, should test weak. Finally, ask the client to repeat the word *yes*. The arm should test strong, while with the word *no* the arm will test weak. This last step is very important to establish rapport with the client's representational systems and with his or her unconscious processes.

Occasionally you will run into a client who exhibits reverse signals, whose arm will respond strong when it should test weak, and vice versa. I find this reversal in one out of every ten persons I work with. Their neuroelectrical systems have been crosswired. Actually, we all experience this crosswiring at one time or another and end up misreading a lot of signals we get from the world. This condition is easily reversed. A person can recover the normal response by thumping on his thymus gland (located at the top of the breastbone) with his fingertips to the count of three, while recalling the image of a loved one. He will then respond strong when tested. Tapping on the thymus gland resets the energy system, bringing it back into correct polarity.

To track an imprint, it must first be energized by recalling the painful event associated with it. A dormant imprint can be very difficult to locate. It is like an inactive program in our computer. When an imprint is energized, the healer can readily detect its whereabouts in the luminous body, as well as the chakra associated with it. Energizing an imprint is like launching a computer program. Its code is activated, and it comes on screen with all of its operations and instructions. To activate an imprint, the client has to recall how she felt at the time she was hurt, remember the pain, sorrow, grief, or shame that she experienced. Intellectual recall is not enough. The client must tap into the intensity of the feelings and experience them viscerally for a few moments.

This test lets the healer determine the presence of a toxic imprint. First test the client's strength by asking her to raise her arm horizontally in front of her and then think of a favorite place in nature. When you press down on her wrist with two fingers, her arm should test strong. Then ask her to recall the painful incident or event that you are evaluating. I ask my clients to close their eyes and become very specific. For example, "Where do you feel the shame [or grief] in your body? Where did you hurt, and how did you hurt when this occurred?" Or I might ask, "Show me with a movement or a posture what it felt like." If my client cannot remember the actual event, I ask her to focus on her feelings at that moment. If an imprint is associated with this incident, her arm will test weak. The difference will be dramatic, as her physical strength will seem to have been drained.

John is a student in our Healing the Light Body School. One morning I was demonstrating this technique and invited him to serve as a subject for the class. As he approached the front of the room, I noticed how muscular he was and how he strutted forward with a show-me attitude. He was not going to allow me to push his arm down no matter how hard I tried. When I asked him to recall a favorite place in nature his arm became like a steel beam. After recalling the pain of his recent divorce and his forced separation from his son, his arm became like putty. He stared at me with a bewildered look on his face, for to him his level of strength had felt unchanged. "Your two fingers felt like a two-hundred-pound lead weight," he said.

The body does not lie. When a client tests positive for an imprint I track to find which chakra comes on-line when the imprint is active. There is always a chakra associated with an active imprint, as there is no other way for the imprint to transfer its information into our nervous system. For example, say that a client's imprint was caused by an experience of neglect in early childhood. If I find the second chakra compromised, I know that this imprint can trigger problems with self-esteem. If the compromised chakra lies in the forehead (the sixth chakra), then I know that the incident has affected my client's ability to discern her life direction, or that she is trying to heal an emotional problem through her intellect.

The healer should test for the chakra linked to an imprint immediately, while the client's Luminous Energy Field is still rippling with the aftershocks of the grief or pain she recalled. I teach my students to bring one hand over the first chakra, two inches above the skin, while the client holds her arm outstretched horizontally as before. Push down on her wrist using the index and middle fingers of your other hand. The procedure is repeated for each of the chakras, beginning with the root and moving up to the crown. I tell my students to pause for one breath in between each chakra, yet proceed quickly, as the ripples caused by the memories of the trauma will diminish rapidly.

Several chakras may test weak, indicating that there are multiple energy centers associated with this imprint. We want to identify the lowest chakra that tests weak, for therein lies the root of the problem. This is the compromised chakra that we want to work with later during the Illumination Process. When this chakra is cleansed and the imprint is erased from the Luminous Energy Field, the higher chakras return to balance by themselves.

We have all lived through painful experiences that did not leave their mark in our Luminous Energy Field. When we process the feelings and emotions at the time a traumatic event occurs, no imprint is etched into the luminous body. When we test these incidents, the client will always test strong. I remember seeing a construction worker who had lost his parents in an auto accident the year before. He had spent many months grieving and was still mourning the loss of his mother and father when we tested for the presence of an imprint. To the surprise of both of us, he tested strong, indicating that there was no imprint in his luminous body associated with this loss. A few weeks earlier, though, he had witnessed a fellow worker slice off his forefinger with a power saw. He recalled how the man had dropped to all fours to find his severed finger in the sawdust as he screamed with pain. This incident so strongly affected my client that he had been unable to work with power tools ever since. When I asked him to recall how he felt when he saw his friend searching for his finger on the ground, I found that his strength abandoned him.

MUSCLE TESTING

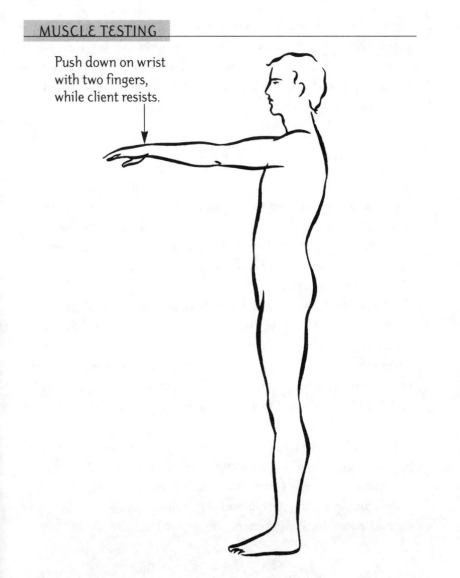

Push down on wrist
with two fingers,
while client resists.

Somehow this incident had imprinted itself in his psyche. After two
Illumination sessions he was able to work again with power tools
without becoming anxious.

Imprints in the Luminous Energy Field can be erased only

through the compromised chakra. They contain pain, grief, or shame that a client may have carried for many years. When I access an imprint through the correct chakra, its emotional landscape begins to reveal itself, and I can sense the wound of origin that caused the imprint in the first place.

Open Sacred Space

It is vital to open a sacred space before beginning the following energy work. The healer may open the space at the start of the day and close it when the last client leaves, or may open the space for each client. Either way client and healer are both safely enveloped in the protected space. Employ the prayer given in Chapter 6 until you discover your own prayer.

The physical space in which you do your work is as important as the energetic space you create. In my office I have calming spiritual elements such as incense, wall hangings, and earth-tone rugs. Two chairs and a sofa provide a seating area for my clients, and at one end of the room I have a massage table covered with a white sheet on which I perform Illuminations. On a low table I have my altar, a collection of stones and ceremonial objects given to me by my teachers. My altar is discreetly placed, as many of my clients are businesspeople who would be uncomfortable with too "mystical" an environment. Nonetheless, my work space is my shaman's cave, and the décor is designed to make my clients feel comfortable and safe, with a sense that they have entered a soothing environment outside their ordinary world.

Envelop Your Client in Your Luminous Energy Field

After creating a sacred space that invites in the natural powers of the directions and its archetypal animals, create an inner sacred space by extending your own Luminous Energy Field over the client. When you call in the directions you create a natural sacred space in which you have access to the organizing principles of nature. When you envelop your client in your Luminous Energy Field, you create a distinctly human sphere, wherein you can access human sources of guidance and knowledge. The first space envelops us in the energies that inform the ecosphere — the natural forces that are healing to the body. The eighth chakra envelops us in the energies that inform the noosphere — the light beings and illuminated masters that we work with.

When I practice the Illumination Process I always open both the natural and human sacred spaces. We want to be informed by the forces that shape the galaxies and the grasses, as well as by the spiritual wisdom that guides our human experience. When we do this we are in twice-sacred space. My client feels as if she is resting in a womblike sphere.

To start, use the Invocation in Chapter 6, then expand your eighth chakra over yourself and your client, enveloping her in a blanket of light for the duration of the session. The client lies faceup, either on the floor or on a massage table. The healer sits directly behind the client's head. The massage table I use is only eighteen inches off the floor, allowing me to sit comfortably in a chair behind her head. I ask the client to inhale through her nose and exhale through her mouth, allowing her breath to find its own rhythm. At a certain point her breath will become faster or slower on its own. The breath regulates the speed of combustion of the energies in the chakra. It is like stoking a fire. By slowing or speeding the breath the client can regulate the intensity of her own process. Sometimes you might ask the client to follow your breathing to help her breath find its own pace. You should turn your face slightly to the side during this process so that you are not breathing directly on the client.

APPLY DEEPENING POINTS

Next cradle the client's head in both of your hands while holding the pressure points in the back of her head. These points, known in

DEEPENING AND RELEASE POINTS

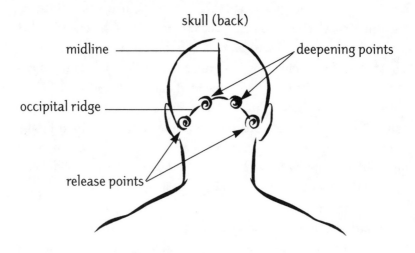

skull (back)

midline

deepening points

occipital ridge

release points

acupuncture as the heavenly gate, help to bring the client into a light trance. They are located at the base of the skull, underneath the occipital ridge. When you cradle a client's head, your hands naturally go to this spot. Gently reach underneath the client's skull. When you apply pressure to these two points, the client enters into a deep state of relaxation within minutes. With your two middle fingers about an inch apart from the midline of the skull, exert gentle, firm pressure. Be sure the client's head remains relaxed and resting on a firm pillow. Hold the deepening points for at least ten minutes. During this time I ask my client in a soft, barely audible voice what she is experiencing. You need to maintain an open line of communication with the client so that she can give you feedback on her process. The client's pupils may begin to move beneath her closed eyelids. This rapid eye movement, or REM, usually denotes a dream state, but in the Illumination Process it denotes a light trance in which the censoring, critical mind has relaxed its grip on consciousness. Some persons report feeling as if they are in a deep sleep, but one where they can speak freely with the healer. They become witnesses to the energetic process and can observe it without being overwhelmed by it.

OPEN THE CHAKRA

Synchronize your breathing with your client's. After holding the deepening points for several minutes, reach down and open the compromised chakra by holding one hand a few inches over your client's chakra, sensing the swirling energy of the disk, and then rotating your hand counterclockwise three or four times. (Sometimes I use an eagle feather for this process, as it allows me to reach the lower chakras without leaving my place by my client's head.) If you have a long reach, you can use your fingers to open a lower chakra; otherwise move to the client's side, letting go of her head while you perform this step, and then immediately return to your position at the head of the table. Whichever method you use, focus your attention carefully.

As soon as the chakra is opened, it begins to "backwash" — to release its sludge and toxic energies. These energies stream out into the large luminous sphere created by the healer's eighth chakra, where they are combusted. I often perceive dark streamers, like thick ribbons, swirling out of the chakra. Respin the chakra counterclockwise several times over the next few minutes, since it can become clogged when it backwashes. Check in with your client to see how she is feeling. Sometimes my clients report a change in body temperature, involuntary muscle spasms, or spontaneous jerking and electrical-like discharges throughout their body. This is a sign that energies around the imprint are being combusted and expelled. Spontaneous body movements occur when muscular and cellular memories are released. When the energy of an imprint has been somatized, that is, assimilated into body tissue, it can only be cleared by this spontaneous, sometimes uncontrollable movement. This is often the case when there was physical trauma in the original wounding, such as incidents of physical abuse, because the body tissues hold memories of these events. In certain cases, a client can begin to thrash about like a fish out of water and hurt herself. It is important to pace the process by speeding up or slowing the breath so the release remains gentle.

I remind my clients that they can slow down or stop the process at any time by crossing their arms over their chest.

Apply Release Points

This process should be done for five minutes, and it is crucial not to overlook it. Applying the release points completes the discharge of heavy energies from the imprint and the sludge in the chakra. Clearing the energy in a clogged chakra is like cleaning your water pipes. Clearing the energy around an imprint is like cleaning the spring your drinking water comes from. You achieve this when you apply the release points. The release points are located at the back of the skull, halfway behind the ears and the midline of the head. Find them on your head right now, reaching with your fingers about three inches behind the ears. They protrude like knobs on the occipital ridge. When held gently, these points trigger the deep clearing, so that the energies enfolding the imprint are dislodged and can be combusted.

Extract Dense Energies

Sometimes an imprint will release sludge that is too dense to combust easily. I sense these energies like blobs of oil inside the chakra. You can gather these thick energies with your hand as you spin the chakra counterclockwise. Flick these energies into the ground with a quick snap of your wrist. The Earth mulches these energies back into life in the same way that it mulches leaves into compost.

CALL ON JAGUAR

I call on the spirit of jaguar to assist in metabolizing heavy energies. When I call on jaguar I can feel a large jungle cat, black as the night, enter into the space and consume the toxic energies being released. Jaguar is the great mulcher that transforms death back into life. At this stage the client will experience the most intense physical sensations, because energy is moving rapidly throughout her body. Some clients report sensations like bolts of lightning shooting up and down their spine. Gradually the client's breath will become very still, signaling that the release stage of the process is complete.

ILLUMINATE TO CLEAR THE IMPRINT

Now the healer performs the Illumination. I recognize this stage of the process, because my client reaches a state of natural resolution. You may notice a palpable shift in the energy. The intensity diminishes, and there is a pervading sense of peace. Place your hand over the open chakra to check that it is spinning smoothly and evenly. Then reach above your head with your right hand, gathering the energy of your eighth chakra and bringing it down into the client's open chakra. I visualize a radiant sun above my head and see my hand gathering scoops of sunlight and showering the chakra with this golden light. I repeat this step three times. The Illumination overwrites the imprint with pure light.

BALANCE THE CHAKRA AND CLOSE THE LUMINOUS ENERGY FIELD

After the Illumination, bring your hands once again to the base of the client's occipital ridge and hold the deepening points for several minutes. This helps the client to relax while the luminous body establishes a new, healed architecture. The client might experience physical twitching and small energy discharges during this phase. Now balance the chakra by spinning it three or four times in a clockwise direction. Next close your own Luminous Energy Field, gathering it back until it becomes a luminous orb above your head.

The expanded Luminous Energy Field is the combustion chamber for burning heavy energies. When you close your field, you dim these fires and contain them within the eighth chakra, where they become pure light. I have seen healers who neglected to close their own field after an Illumination absorb toxic energies from their client, and become ill themselves.

Process with the Client

Invite your client to sit up when he is ready, and ask him to share his experience. Everyone experiences the Illumination Process in their own way. Some clients report physical sensations almost exclusively, everything from twitching or energy streaming up and down their legs to tingling in their extremities. Others are more attuned to the imagery that spontaneously appears during the process. Still others report only a deep sense of relaxation, or feeling as though they have been asleep.

The Illumination Process heals both physical and psychological conditions. When the toxic energies around an imprint are cleared, the body's immune response is disinhibited and physical healing is accelerated. Psychological conditions are drained of their energy when their imprints are no longer operant. Many times the healing is nearly spontaneous.

Close the Directions

When we open sacred space we create a microcosm that spans across the visible and invisible worlds. The forces that sustain the daffodils and the spiral arms of galaxies are present within it. When we close sacred space we release these natural forces and the archetypal power animals to return to their undifferentiated state. You close sacred space by turning again to the four directions, starting with the South and working clockwise, thanking each of the archetypal animals for being with you. Do the same for Heaven and Earth. You can blow scented water or sage smoke as you do this. If a shaman feels she needs to send one of the archetypal animals home with her client, she will leave that direction open, asking the archetype to look after and heal her client.

CHAPTER 8

THE EXTRACTION PROCESS

He just doubled up and fell forward on his medicine objects. I was assisting others in our group. They were starting their vision quests at Amaru Machay, an initiation cave decorated with carvings of serpents and jaguars. It was eleven o'clock at night, and I heard Eduardo calling faintly. When I reached him he was frothing at the mouth. I thought that he was having a seizure.

"They've gotten me, compadre,*" he whispered between halting breaths. He was sweating profusely, even though the night was cool. He told me he had been struck by black magic in the middle of the ceremony. The hair on the back of my neck stood on end. Eduardo is a renowned shaman from the North Coast of Peru. I have known him for years and know his power. How could anyone successfully attack this man? I know that there are many people envious of the attention that the Peruvian media accords him. Even the president of the country has consulted him.*

"I've been stabbed," he said. He indicated that a dagger had been thrust into his shoulder, nearly striking his heart. I could see nothing there. I reached for the bottle of flower essences in his altar, took a mouthful of it, and placed my lips on his shoulder. I could feel a metallic taste in my mouth. I began to suck out this object, feeling nausea come over me. Suddenly the knifelike object broke loose and entered my mouth. I could feel it going down past my trachea and into my stomach. I began to retch

uncontrollably. I couldn't stop emptying my gut, until all I had left were the dry heaves.

Eduardo, sat up, regaining his composure. "Thank you, compadre," he said. "You saved my life."

It's been two days since this incident, and I can still feel the ache in my stomach. That's the last time I'm doing a sucking extraction.

JOURNALS

It could have happened only in Brazil. What an eclectic mix of Indian, European, and African — all of the shades of color imaginable in people. There was an international business conference at the hotel next to ours. At the beach that evening it occurred to me that evolution had taken a fork somewhere. At one end were the Brazilians, whose shapely, graceful bodies seemed to float above Ipanema beach. At the other end of the strand the pale, overweight conventioneers lay like beached walruses, holding exotic drinks with little umbrellas in them.

You can be anything you want in Brazil — even a medical doctor initiated in the Afro-Brazilian traditions. Last night I took my group to visit this doctor. He has a group of highly trained mediums, expert trackers who would incorporate a former lifetime of the client's in order to heal it. Minutes after Esther, one of the women in my group, lay down, one of the mediums began to sob and wail, saying in a little girl's voice, "Don't touch me. Please, don't touch me anymore."

Esther's sister was with us on this journey and looked at me bewildered. She had no idea what was going on. Then another medium went into trance and claimed to be Esther's deceased brother. He turned to Esther and said that he could not find peace until she forgave him. He began to apologize for hurting her, for abusing her when she was little. I turned to Esther's sister and asked her what was going on. Dumbfounded, she explained to me that their brother, who had died a year earlier, had repeatedly molested Esther when she was young.

Esther sat up and began comforting the medium who was sobbing like a child, while speaking to her deceased brother. The brother said he was in pain, and that he was sorry he had hurt her. They carried on talking for close to twenty minutes. At the end of this Esther said to her brother: "I forgive you. Go in peace. I love you." At that point, as if by clockwork, the two mediums disengaged and sat up as if nothing had happened. They had no recollection of what had taken place. One of the mediums had incorporated the spirit of Esther the child, while the other had incorporated the spirit of the departed brother who had been hovering around Esther since he died, seeking to be forgiven. Only in Brazil.

JOURNALS

THE MAXIM THAT NO MAN IS AN ISLAND IS QUITE TRUE. AS A PART of the larger world body, we are all connected. We know that the electromagnetic component of the Luminous Energy Field expands away from the body at the speed of light. One's energy field overlaps with the energy fields of everyone else. Imagine dropping a pebble into a still pool and seeing the ripples spread outward from the center. Now imagine dropping another pebble into the pool. The ripples caused by these two pebbles overlap and soon intersect, creating the same interference patterns in the water that our energy fields create in space. We interact energetically with each other all the time.

EXTRACTING CRYSTALLIZED ENERGIES

While the Illumination Process combusts most energies in the Luminous Energy Field, some toxic energies can crystallize, becoming nearly material objects, which are impossible to metabolize through the Illumination Process. They are like petrified wood, which no longer burns. These crystallized energies embed themselves in the physical body, taking on shapes such as daggers, arrows, spears, and swords. Amazon shamans believe that crystallized energies are the result of black magic or sorcery. I have found that these energies can be caused by anger, envy, or hatred directed at us by another person. Sometimes they are also energetic remnants—memories of how we died, how we were hurt, or how we were killed in a former existence.

Obviously, our family, friends, and associates—the people who are closest to us—have the greatest potential for bringing joy and causing pain in our lives. Their direct access to our most private selves makes us vulnerable to their betrayal, anger, or jealousy. A negative thought from an angry former spouse can penetrate our luminous body like a dagger. When they first enter us, these energies travel through the Luminous Energy Field. Our system recognizes these energies as foreign and generally will eradicate them in the same way the immune system eliminates foreign bacteria. However, when we are under a continual barrage of negativity, the defense systems of the luminous body can become overwhelmed. Negative energy directed toward us can crystallize and embed itself in the physical body. This happens over a period of weeks or months. These energies do not belong to us. Because the energy has become nearly material, it must be extracted manually. The extraction must take place only after an Illumination has cleared a client's Luminous Energy Field.

I observed one version of the Extraction Process in the headwaters of the Amazon, where I had been studying with a jungle shaman. Her client that evening was a storekeeper, an influential man from a nearby town. He had traveled three days into the rain forest to see the medicine woman. He complained that for the last few months he had felt lethargic, experienced continual digestive problems, and lost his appetite. On top of that, his relationship with his family had deteriorated and his wife was threatening to leave him.

The shaman asked the shopkeeper to lie down. She summoned the four directions and packed her medicine pipe with *huaman sayre* tobacco, the visionary tobacco of the upper Amazon. She struck a match, brought it to the pipe bowl, inhaled deeply, and offered a prayer to Mother Earth, followed by another prayer to Father Sky. She blew smoke across the man's outstretched form, scanning his luminous body in the bluish cloud. Every now and again she passed her hand over his body. When she finished, she asked him to sit up. The medicine woman diagnosed his condition as a case of *daño*, or black magic caused by envy.

Next, the medicine woman cradled the man's head, singing softly and cleansing his Luminous Energy Field by stroking it with a fan made from macaw feathers. All along the shopkeeper complained of a pain over his abdomen. The shaman stated matter-of-factly that a spear was stuck in his side. A man that he had helped was betraying him, she said. He was taking advantage of his kindness, and consorting with his wife when he traveled. She then reached down to his belly, wrapped her hand around an invisible shaft, and began tugging at it. She held one hand firmly against his belly and pulled at the invisible spear shaft with her other hand, turning and twisting it, gently dislodging it. By now the man was moaning, saying that he felt as if a spike were being pulled out of his abdomen. At the end of the treatment the shopkeeper lay on the grass mat, exhausted. The shaman continued to counsel him. It was important to be generous and giving, she said, but it was equally as important not to be foolish. The spear that she had wrenched from his abdomen was caused by the jealousy that this other man had of his success.

When I asked the medicine woman why she had performed an energy cleansing prior to the extraction, she explained that the heavy energies around the shaft needed to be combusted before the spear could be removed. Even though these energies were not solid like the shaft, they held it firmly in place, like the dirt packed around a stake driven into the ground. The medicine woman might have performed a sucking extraction, which is commonly practiced in the Amazon. This was dangerous, as she might accidentally swallow the energy and become ill herself. The two-step Illumination and Extraction Process is much safer.

At first I thought that the Amazon shamans perceived daggers, spears, and arrows embedded in their clients because such objects were the stuff of their everyday lives. When I returned home I expected to find objects that conformed more or less to the symbols of modern warfare — guns and bullets — embedded in the Luminous Energy Field of my clients. To my surprise, I found exactly the same symbols that the jungle healers described. I could make no sense of this until I considered that the brain's limbic system evolved thousands of years ago at a time when our ancestors hunted game and slew each other with knives and spears. The repertoire of images of this ancient brain structure remained unchanged.

The limbic brain takes the symbolic as literal. When we have been betrayed, we say that we have been "stabbed in the back" because symbolically we have. Such traitorous acts and the intense emotions that accompany them create pools of stagnant energy in the Luminous Energy Field. The longer it takes for one to recover from this betrayal, the more time this energy has to crystallize. Eventually, it begins to acquire the shape of a dagger stuck in one's back, as this is the way that our limbic brain perceives it. When we suffer from heartbreak, these energies can assume the shape of a metal band constricting the heart, or a steel trap that has our feelings locked in its grip. Likewise, sexual abuse during a client's early years often appears as an arrow or shaft piercing the lower belly, puncturing the chakra where sexuality and self-esteem reside. Once I found an energetic noose around the neck of a client who had been choking in her abusive marriage.

It is important to remain open-minded with this work. When I feel a dense cylindrical object in my client's body, I don't immediately think, Ah, *spear!* Instead, I note my sensations, saying to myself,

Warm, cylindrical, long, rigid..., and so on. I only conclude that the object must be a knife when I have extracted it and found that indeed it has a sharp blade and a handle. I encourage my students to avoid naming what they feel, as naming is a rational act that separates us from the experience. I caution my students not to extract crystallized energies until they have mastered the Illumination Process. Students in the Healing the Light Body School learn to develop a fine kinesthetic sense to accurately feel for crystallized energies. At the beginning it is easy to confuse the dense energies that gather around an imprint for an embedded energy.

CRYSTALLIZED ENERGIES FROM FORMER LIFETIMES

In the course of my work with medicine people, I learned that crystallized energies that have hardened within the body often originate from former lifetimes. They have been within us for so long that they have become embedded in body tissue. During an extraction clients will spontaneously describe images from a different era — the field of battle where they were abandoned to die, or their homes being burned and relatives slain.

Patricia was a successful attorney in Chicago when she came to see me. She was nearly fifty years old and had never been in a love relationship that lasted for more than a few months. She had a sexual addiction and had been undergoing psychological treatment for some time. "I use men like Kleenexes," Patricia said to me when we first met. She described herself as losing interest in men after she made love with them. She couldn't bring herself to spend the entire night with a lover and would send him home after having sex. She had been involved with more than a dozen men in the last year but found fault with every one and soon dropped them. She had been referred to me by her therapist, who felt that she was not making any progress with Patricia.

During the Illumination Process, I thought that there might be a crystallized energy involved. When I scanned her Luminous Energy Field, I sensed a number of narrow, shaftlike objects protruding from her heart. They felt like porcupine quills, and when I scanned closely I sensed her heart was like a pincushion. I returned to the release points at the base of the skull and gently held these. When the release points are triggered, they reveal the full landscape of a chakra, with all of its stories and players.

When I moved my hands back to her chest I again sensed numerous cold, metallic quills projecting from her heart. When I touch these crystallized energies their memories are activated. I grabbed hold of one of the quills, and Patricia reported an image of a young man in his late teens living in the rain forest. He was part of a band of peaceful native people who fished and gathered the abundant fruit available. She saw a group of men gathered in a clearing where his family had set up camp. All the huts had been set on fire, and she could smell the stench of burning flesh. Patricia then began seeing from the perspective of the young man. As he drew closer he saw that the men were molesting his younger sister. The boy strung an arrow on his bow and let it fly. His arrow pierced the rapist through the neck. Immediately the rest of the men gave chase and caught him. Patricia was describing the scene in great detail, seeing it like a movie playing itself out before her. She saw how the boy was gang-raped by the thugs who had killed his family. Afterward he was tied to a tree and left to die of starvation. Patricia could feel the rage and disgust the young man experienced. And she carried the same rage against men whom she used for sex. The porcupine quills that I perceived were her defense system against becoming intimate with anyone.

As I extracted the quill-like objects, Patricia sobbed and pounded her fist angrily on the floor. I then performed an Illumination to change the affinities that attracted these energies. When we discussed the images she had seen during her healing, Patricia felt that she had been this young man and that this experience made her disgusted with men in general. It is difficult to say with certainty whether the images of a boy being gang-raped were indeed from one of Patricia's former lives. Whether it was a previous incarnation or a metaphor for her life today did not much matter. This was a story that lived within her and informed her life. Dozens of psychological interpretations exist for the images Patricia perceived. These explanations, however, do not detract from the real benefits that Patricia received from her healing. Shortly thereafter she began dating a man on a regular basis. Her promiscuity ended. Her therapist called me a few months later to tell me that Patricia was making progress in understanding her complex dynamics around intimacy.

One of my favorite examples of the power of the Extraction Process is my own. While playing on the beach with my nine-year-old son, I had just lifted him onto my shoulders when a wave knocked both of us down, and he landed on my upturned arm. I tore the rotator cuff in my right shoulder. This painful condition prevented me from lifting my right arm above my head. Six months of physical therapy had no effect, and my doctor suggested that I consider surgery.

As I was teaching the Extraction Process during our Healing the Light Body program, it occurred to me that the process might help my shoulder. I asked one of our senior faculty, Dr. Richard Jones, to scan my shoulder for crystallized energy. Richard examined my Luminous Energy Field and informed me that he sensed an object protruding from my armpit. He described a metallic piece extending about four inches beyond the skin. After enveloping me in his Luminous Energy Field, he performed an Illumination. In the middle of the Illumination, he instructed me to sit up, and proceeded to extract the metallic piece. As he turned the object, I felt a pain shooting all the way to my fingertips and spreading into the side of my neck. It felt as if a knife blade were being twisted inside my scapula. I followed the pain as it traveled through the inside of my shoulder. It took close to five minutes for Richard to extract the embedded object, which was shaped like a dagger with a triangular handle.

My rotator cuff healed within a month, and I recovered full range of motion. During the process I perceived no images or clues about the origin of this energy. Richard believed it was an ancient wound associated with a loss I had suffered, but he could give me no further details. I was convinced that this was an energetic residue from a sucking extraction I had performed years earlier on Don Eduardo. Richard encouraged me to remain open to later interpretation. I recognized the theme of loss in my life, yet could not relate it to any current or past trauma. Often a client does not perceive or recall any images during the Extraction Process, although images may come days or weeks later in dreams or reverie. I continued to mull over the idea of loss. Although Richard is a clinical psychologist, he did not press me to make sense of my experience too quickly, nor to attach a story of past-life trauma to my healing. After a time, the story revealed itself to me in a dream. I was riding on horseback through a dark wood. The farther I went, the darker the forest became. I could sense the trail becoming narrower, until the branches made further going impossible. There was no room to turn the horse, and I could go no deeper into the wood. Then a tall woman in a blue robe appeared. She took hold of the reins and said I had to continue home on foot. When I tried to dismount, I noticed I had lost the use of my right arm, which hung limply by my side. She had to help me down and lead me out of the forest, and I leaned on her for support. When I woke up I understood that the dream was telling me I had to integrate a missing element of the feminine into my life. I could not rely on the right arm, the masculine side, to bring me home safely. When I mentioned this dream to Richard he commented that my interpretation felt right. He did not impose his analysis on me. In our work, the client discovers the stories that result in his own healing.

EXTRACTING HARDENED ENERGIES

The technique that follows is used to draw out energies that have crystallized in the physical body. The Extraction Process consists of several steps that include scanning the client's Luminous Energy Field and identifying and extracting the crystallized energy. Always perform the Extraction Process during an Illumination. Unless the crystallized energy lies at the outermost layer of the Luminous Energy Field, it can be difficult to perceive. During an Illumination the energetic landscape of a chakra reveals itself, and crystallized energies at all levels of the Luminous Energy Field can be easily detected. Moreover, the Illumination Process combusts the energies that collect around the crystallization and keep it wedged into the body. The Illumination is the equivalent of cleaning the dirt from a wound before removing the shards of glass embedded in the skin.

Negative energies are initially attracted to us because they have an affinity with us. We have receptor sites for them the same way that the brain has receptor sites for certain chemicals. We draw these energies to us in the same way that we attract certain kinds of people to ourselves. Every form of energy has a frequency and a vibration. Anger can penetrate our Luminous Energy Field only when the vibration for anger lives within us, and hatred can affect us only when self-hatred is present. A current situation in which negative energy is directed at you — such as a divorce, a bitter feud, or a great disappointment — can create an affinity. Consequently it is not enough to extract the crystallized energies affecting your client. Their affinities have to be changed — the self-hatred or anger healed — so that the client does not attract a similar energy once again. The Illumination Process heals a client's affinities for these energies by clearing and stepping up the frequency at which a chakra spins. As the vibratory rate of a chakra increases, we begin to attract pure, clear, beneficent energies.

After performing an Illumination but before closing the chakra, a healer performs the Extraction Process. There are five steps to this process, which takes about twenty minutes to perform.

1. Scan the Luminous Energy Field.
2. Tease out heavy energy.
3. Apply release points.
4. Extract the object.
5. Illuminate the chakra.

SCAN THE LUMINOUS ENERGY FIELD

Make passes with your hand a few inches above the client's body, as if you are stroking her energy field—going slowly, feeling for sensations of heat or cold. Variations in temperature often indicate the presence of a crystallized energy. When you sense a shape, wrap your hand around it and try to obtain an impression. Does it feel like metal, wood, or stone? Try to avoid naming what you feel; rather, stay with the sensations.

TEASE OUT HEAVY ENERGY

Next tease out the heavy energy at the base of the object, gathering these energies with your fingertips and flicking them to the Earth. This begins to loosen the embedded object.

APPLY RELEASE POINTS

Then hold the release points at the back of the skull, to trigger the release of any remaining toxic energies in the chakra. There may not be a linear relationship between the site of the crystallized energy and the compromised chakra. It is possible to find an embedded energy in the feet that involves the heart chakra.

EXTRACT THE OBJECT

Draw out the object, gently moving it from side to side and twisting to loosen it. Invite the client to bring her awareness to the site and to feel your actions, asking her, "Am I going too fast? Too slow? Is it painful?" You may also ask the client to report what images she perceives.

ILLUMINATE THE CHAKRA

Illuminate the chakra, bathing it in pure light, to increase its vibratory rate and change the affinity. Finally close the chakra and process with the client.

It is important to sense with your hands during the Extraction Process. Even though I'm primarily a visual person and I see these crystallized energies, I carefully scan my client's Luminous Energy Field with my hands. Imagine your tactile sense becoming so heightened that you can perceive the tides of energy flowing through the luminous body. Remember that the skin is the largest sensory organ we have. As my students develop their skills, their tactile sense becomes heightened. I teach my students to trust their uncommon sense. Many report being unable to see energies but develop a very fine tactile aptitude. Touch is uncensored. What we feel is private, intimate, and intrinsic to us. This allows us to track precisely for crystallized energies.

INTRUSIVE ENERGIES AND ENTITIES

A crystallized energy embeds itself within the body. An intrusive entity embeds itself within the central nervous system. Intrusive energies and entities cannot be extracted using the technique described above for crystallized energies, since they are fluid and can move around with the body. It is like trying to grasp water; there is simply no way to hold on to it. Many psychological and physical problems are caused or exacerbated by intrusive entities. They often produce anxiety, depression, addictions, mood swings, and a host of other symptoms. One telltale sign of an intrusive entity is when a client displays a range of mutable psychological symptoms that defy diagnostic categories. Once the intrusive entity is set free the client can more readily change his behavior and often experiences spontaneous healing.

Intrusive entities are disincarnate spirits trapped between this world and the next. Sometimes an intrusive entity may be one of our own former lifetimes that has been awakened from our unconscious and wants to live again, thus vying with our present self for access to our central nervous system. Intrusive entities attach themselves to a chakra and through it connect to the central nervous system, where they enter into a parasitic relationship with the host. They are the energy-sucking "lowlifes" of the Spirit world.

Intrusive energies are fluid. They stream throughout the Luminous Energy Field like a dark, rippling tide. They flow from chakra to chakra, cruising through our nervous system. Intrusive entities are fixed to the particular chakra they feed through. Often an intrusive energy is so powerful that it seems to have a personality, and therefore we believe it must be an entity. At other times an entity appears so weak that you are convinced that you are dealing only with an intrusive energy. When persons who are spiritually open become emotionally unbalanced, they are easy targets for parasitic intrusive entities. These disembodied beings are drawn to the spiritually unwary like moths to a flame. No amount of talk therapy will be effective in dealing with this condition. When these energies are extracted, healing can move forward more rapidly.

All energy has consciousness, even the most basic and primitive, so that an intrusive energy can seem to have a humanlike personality. When a healer tunes in to it she can sense the anger, hatred, or envy belonging to the person that directed their thoughts against her client. There are times that I can tell the difference only when I set this energy free at the fire, which is how we clear our extraction crystals. An intrusive energy dissolves back into nature, since it has no Luminous Energy Field to contain it. It is assimilated into the trees, the stones, and the Earth, where it is mulched. An intrusive entity is carried to the Spirit world by luminous healers. These luminous beings help the confused soul regain consciousness and return to the light.

Intrusive entities are more common than we would like to believe. An intrusive entity may appear as one of two types: one of our former selves (a former lifetime that has awakened from the subconscious mind), or a disincarnate being who has penetrated our Luminous Energy Field. The intrusive entity may be a deceased relative or friend who is coming to us for assistance. When a person dies suddenly in an accident, or under narcotics in the hospital, he can become lost between this world and the next. He is caught in a nightmare that he cannot wake up from. He is not aware that he has died, and comes to us for comfort. We bring him into the safety of our luminous body, in the same way we would take him into our home if he were hurt or suffering. His energy mixes with ours and begins to wreak havoc in our Luminous Energy Field. The person who has died may not have any harmful intent, but his attachment to a living person can be harmful. Sometimes we begin to exhibit the same physical or emotional symptoms that the person suffered before he died. When I extract an intrusive entity from the Luminous Energy Field, my client's physical and psychological symptoms often disappear.

One out of four people who come to see me has been affected by intrusive energies or entities. At times they can be spirits that actually desire to harm my client, perhaps wronged people from another time and place. Intrusive entities feed on the energy of the chakras and central nervous system. There is no more nutritious form of energy. They attach themselves to the spinal cord through one of the chakras and are able to experience that person's thoughts and feelings. The Luminous Energy Field has a difficult time eliminating these foreign energies. Unlike the physical body, which can eliminate the elements it cannot use through urination, bowel movements, sweat, and respiration, the luminous body has no openings. When these energies have entered the central nervous system, we have to extract them using a crystal.

EXTRACTION CRYSTALS

Crystals are the most stable structures in nature. They are transducers, which means that they can convert one kind of energy into another very easily. This is why they are used in electronic chips inside computers. Clear quartz is best for extracting intrusive energies and entities. Quartz is such a stable element that energy is naturally drawn to it. A flawless double-terminated piece of quartz four to five inches long is one of the finest instruments in the healer's medicine bag. These crystals are hand-cut from a piece of nearly perfect, clear quartz, and are expensive. I advise my students to invest in the best possible crystal they can afford. It is important that the extraction crystal be clear and have no surface fractures. When a crystal has fractures, the energy can leak out and contaminate the healer. When the crystal has inclusions, clouds, or intersecting planes, the intrusive entity experiences a great deal of pain when it is inside the crystal. Remember that the entity you are extracting might be a deceased relative or former incarnation of your client. I no more want an intrusive energy/entity to suffer than I want my client to be in pain. As a healer, your mandate is to heal, regardless of which side of the Spirit world your client is in. Their temporary crystal home should be a comfortable and sheltered place, or they will resist being extracted.

After extracting an intrusive entity, I help my client change her affinities, so that she no longer attracts this (or a similar) entity, just as we do for the crystallized energies. We do this again through the Illumination Process. In this case the healer must not only extract the disturbing entity but heal it as well. We can help this lost soul awaken from the nightmare in which it is trapped, and return to the light and love of the Spirit world.

Physicians in Brazil's Spiritist Medical Association have found that up to half of their patient's maladies are caused by a disturbing energy or entity. Six months after the death of my paternal grandmother, I received a research grant to study these physicians, who gathered in São Paulo every Friday evening for spiritual healing sessions. They sat in a circle around a medium — an attractive, dark-skinned woman in her early thirties — who incorporated the spirits of recently deceased patients so that they might regain consciousness long enough to receive healing from the living. My grandmother and I had been very close. I had spent more time with her during my childhood than with my own mother. I had been depressed since her death a few months earlier and thought how wonderful it would be if she could receive this kind of treatment. After two long hours of ministering to the spirits of the departed, the Lord's Prayer was recited to close the healing circle. Suddenly the medium shuddered and went into trance again. She began speaking in Spanish rather than her native Portuguese. The healer in charge resumed the session. No one wanted to let this spirit continue suffering.

"Where am I? God help me," she said in a weak, tremulous voice.

The medium had embodied the spirit of an older woman, disoriented and in pain, who said her lips were dry and cracked from breathing through a respirator tube. She wanted to be allowed to die. One of the physicians in the circle explained to the spirit that she had already died. He explained that she was temporarily occupying the body of a medium and encouraged her to feel the medium's physique.

As her hands moved down her dress, the healer asked, "Are those your hands, your breasts?"

"No, they are young...."

The spirit did not realize that she was dead. She was still in her hospital room, hooked up to breathing and feeding tubes. She had been brought here to be released from a place where she knew neither the joy of the living nor the peace of the dead. As I listened, it certainly sounded as if this spirit was suffering.

At that moment the medium looked at me and gasped. "Alber, is that you, my little one? Help me, help me, please."

I heard this as if in a daze. Only my grandmother called me by that name. The healer then asked the woman to notice the other spirits who were there to help her. She began to call out to her mother, her father, her husband — my grandfather. I was speechless. One of the physicians explained to her that she was now leaving the nightmarish realm between the worlds and waking into the world of Spirit, into the light, where she was being greeted by her loved ones. In the Spirit world one could be any age one wanted, as the soul is ageless. The spirit said that her pain and discomfort were leaving her, that she felt younger and stronger.

Before she left she said: "Thank you for bringing me here." Then she turned to me and said, "I will always be with you, Alber."

No one there knew about my grandmother María Luisa or her death. I like to think that she was really with me and that she was assisted in her transition from this world to the next. Within a week, my depression lifted. Later one of the healers explained to me that in her confusion, my grandmother's spirit had attached itself to me, seeking refuge with the person she had the greatest affinity with in our family. My being spiritually open made it so much easier for her to find solace with me. I sensed her suffering, which I experienced as depression and loss of interest in life.

Intrusive entities are seldom dark or evil spirits. They are mostly lost souls seeking healing whatever way they can. But there are exceptions. Occasionally you encounter what I refer to as a "nasty." We will discuss how to deal with these later. As with my grandmother, these are often relatives who come to us for assistance. A rule of thumb is that the greater the number of people who come to you for help in this world, the greater the number of spirits who will seek you out for assistance from the other side. Most of these never penetrate our Luminous Energy Field, as we have no affinities or emotional connection to them. When they do penetrate our luminous defenses, we are helpless. We lack the spiritual technologies that you can find in the traditional cultures of Brazil, the Amazon, or Tibet to assist them.

A shaman once commented to me that he believed Westerners did not bury their dead. I asked him why he thought such a preposterous thing, and he responded that behind each of us were scores of what he called the "undead." These were ancestors who had not been properly mourned after their death. This occurs not because we do not care about them, but simply because we do not possess the knowledge of what happens to the soul after death. We will address this process in detail in the next chapter. The irony is that when we do not honor and mourn our ancestors, they continue living through us. They die with a great deal of unresolved business in this world.

EXTRACTING INTRUSIVE ENTITIES AND ENERGIES

For the Illumination Process and most other energy work, one healer works with a client. However, for extracting intrusive energies/ entities, it is best to have two trackers assist the healer. Most of us do not have the luxury of having two trackers assist us in this process, and have to learn to perform all of these functions simultaneously. We have to run energy, track, and extract all at the same time. With practice the healer can master the art. Be sure your client has previously received an Illumination. There are seven steps to this process, which takes about thirty minutes to perform.

1. Test for an intrusive energy/entity.
2. Run energy through the client to dislodge the energy/entity.
3. Track the energy/entity in the client's body.
4. Extract the energy/entity.

5. Process with the client.
6. Perform an Illumination to change affinities and complete the healing.
7. Cleanse the crystal to release the energy/entity.

Test for an Intrusive Energy/Entity

We use the muscle-testing procedure described in Chapter 7 to ascertain if there is an intrusive entity or energy present. I have my client stand up, clasp his hands together, and hold his arms before him, parallel to the ground. I then ask him to resist as I try to push his arms down, exerting pressure on his wrist with my right hand. The level of strength I find during the muscle testing will be the benchmark for the state of the client's Luminous Energy Field.

Run Energy through the Client

Stand behind the client with your dominant hand at the base of her spine, over the coccyx. Your other hand rests at the base of the neck. Since I am right-handed, I place my right hand at the base of the spine and the left at the base of the neck. Left-handed people may reverse this. Run energy between your hands, from the bottom to the top. I visualize red-hot energy flowing through my client's spine. Run the energy for several minutes until you feel it streaming through the spine and into your hand at the client's neck. This fire-hot energy temporarily dislodges any intrusive energy/entity attached to the spinal cord.

When you feel the energy is flowing strongly, retest your client. If the client's strength is as great or greater than the benchmark level, no energy/entity is present and no Extraction is necessary. If their strength level is substantially weaker than the benchmark, an Extraction is needed. When an energy/entity is dislodged from the central nervous system, the strength of the Luminous Energy Field momentarily collapses. Physical strength leaves for a moment as well. When there is no intrusive energy/entity, the Luminous Energy Field is strengthened by the energy the healer is running through the client's central nervous system.

TRACK THE ENERGY/ENTITY

If the healer has two assistants, the healer will be doing the Extraction while one of the assistants is tracking and the other is running energy. The person running energy sends it up the client's spine in both the testing process and the actual Extraction. The tracker locates and monitors the position of the energy/entity during the process. As this energy/entity is fluid, it can migrate to different chakras and up or down the spine. The extractor will need an extraction crystal, which should be double-terminated, as clear as possible, and ideally four or five inches long.

The tracker stands beside the client, placing one hand on her shoulder and the other hand on her waist. The energy runner begins to direct energy along the client's spine. As the extractor, the healer stands in front of the client, facing her. The client's hands are hanging freely by her sides. Holding the crystal in one of his palms, the healer takes hold of the client's hands in his. The healer then begins to jiggle the client's hands, moving them up and down while simultaneously tuning in to the energy/entity. The healer takes his time with this process, using his breathing to remain calm and centered. He asks the client to report any feelings or images that she perceives.

EXTRACT THE ENERGY/ENTITY

The actual extraction must be performed within five minutes after energizing the spine, before the intrusive energy/entity readheres to it. The healer continues to jiggle the client's arms and begins to draw the energy/entity down into his own hands. He waits for a signal from the runner that the energy is flowing strongly along the spine. Then the tracker tells him where she perceives the intrusion. She monitors the energy/entity as it is dislodged from the spine and moves on to another chakra or attempts to hide within the client's body. Often the intrusion realizes that it is being extracted and does its best to cling to its host. The tracker monitors the progress and gives the healer feedback on location and intensity.

My task as a healer performing the Extraction Process is to coax out the energy/entity. I know that it is scared and confused. I talk to it silently, and at times out loud, telling it that it is going to be safe, that it will be looked after, that it is not going to suffer any longer, and that everything is going to be all right. I tell it that I am here to help it heal, and reassure it that it will come to no harm. I often speak to the energy/entity as I do to a very young child. I understand that it is suffering, and I want to help alleviate its pain. As I coax it out, I feel the energy entering my forearms. I do not allow the energy to travel past my elbows. (Even if the healer has no affinities for the energy, it can affect his Luminous Energy Field.) As soon as I feel it coming out of my client, I draw it out into the crystal.

There are times when the energy/entity will refuse to leave the client. At other times the client is reluctant to let the intrusive entity go. The client might unconsciously recognize it as a relative, or one of his own former lifetimes, and not want to release it. In these cases I use a startle response. I ask the client to count backward from twenty or to recite the alphabet backward — anything that will distract his rational mind. When I feel the energy/entity begin to move into my forearm, I shout "Ha!" and yank my hands together, capturing the energy/entity in the crystal. I then ask the tracker for feedback. Was the extraction complete? Is another pass necessary? Is there more than one energy/entity? The healer may want to muscle-test again to confirm that the extraction was successful.

Claire is a nurse from Canada who enrolled in our Healing the Light Body School. One day she requested that I demonstrate the

Extraction Process with her. I was reluctant, as I did not sense any problems. Claire was a balanced person, happily married with two children. Every aspect of her life was working to her satisfaction. I wanted to demonstrate with someone I suspected was suffering from an intrusive energy. Nevertheless, she insisted, and I agreed. To my surprise, she tested positive. As I began the extraction, Claire began to shake, and her knees turned to jelly. The person running the energy behind her had to hold her upright, and she became limp like a rag doll. As I was drawing out the energy, Claire bolted upright and screamed "No! I know that this is a trick!" Then she doubled over and began sobbing uncontrollably. I sensed a dark, repulsive energy entering my arms, and yanked it into the crystal, yelling loudly. Claire collapsed to the ground.

Afterward her entire complexion changed. She explained to the class that her father had died four years earlier and that she felt she had been carrying him around ever since. After the extraction she felt drained and had to lie down until the evening, when we released the intrusive energy/entity at the fire. I asked Claire to say any final farewell or goodbye she wanted to express to her father. I had no way of being certain that the energy I had extracted was indeed her father. I was relying on Claire's hunch, and if she was right, I knew that it would be important for her to achieve closure with her departed father. Claire spoke tenderly to the entity while she held the crystal, turning it over in her hands, and related to her dad how much she missed him, how she had never gotten to really know him, and how grateful she was for all her childhood memories. We then released the intrusive energy/entity. I noticed how the space around the fire began to shimmer, and a warm breeze wafted through the cool evening air. Both of these signs indicated to me that a space between the worlds was opening. I could feel the presence of luminous beings, medicine people from the Spirit world, which come to assist a suffering soul. The intrusive entity was received with great love and taken home.

It took Claire nearly a week to recover her strength. During this time she said she felt a joy coming back to her that she had not felt since her father passed away.

If the healer must perform an Extraction Process without assistants, she will have to carry out all tasks by herself. Once the energy is flowing along the spine, the healer moves to the front of her client's body and proceeds with the Extraction. This is where I have to be very mindful, as I have to track and extract at the same time. I engage my kinesthetic sense (touch) so that I can feel the energy descending into my arms and into the crystal. I dialogue with my client and with the energy/entity and track the energy as it moves through my client's body. A healer can learn to perform these tasks at the same time, but it requires practice and can be very draining. I teach students to master each of these tasks separately, working as part of a team of three. Then they can combine these skills when they have to perform an Extraction alone. If, however, I discover that the intrusive energy/entity is a "nasty" that will not exit on its own without putting up a struggle, I always call on two other healers to assist me, one to run energy and one to track.

PROCESS WITH THE CLIENT

I always describe to my client what I perceived when I was tracking the energy/entity, and any information the energy/entity offered me. The questions I generally ask an energy/entity are: Where did it come from? How long has it been with my client? What attracted the energy/entity to my client? What did it want from her? Students sometimes ask me how one can speak with energy. Does energy have a voice? For the shaman, everything in nature has a voice — the rivers, the trees, and energy. I also want to know what my client experienced. How does she feel now? What affinity does she have for this intrusion? Why was it drawn to her in the first place? What needs to be done to prevent a similar problem in the future?

PERFORM AN ILLUMINATION TO COMPLETE THE HEALING

A second Illumination should always follow an Extraction. This changes any affinity for the energy/entity and completes the healing. If the affinity isn't changed, another intrusive energy/entity will seek the client out. An Extraction is a bit like a divorce. You can throw the bum out, but unless you change your affinities, you will end up marrying another. There is no negotiation possible with an intrusive energy/entity, no possible way to learn to live with each other. There is only one humane place for it to go — to nature, or to the Spirit world. When an intrusive entity is a loved one in need of assistance, I ask my client what unresolved issues he still has to heal with this relative. I want to help him discover what his role in the play is, and why he signed up for that part in the first place. This is the time for saying "I love you" and "I forgive you." When the affinity is changed, the client will be unmolested in the future.

CLEANSE THE CRYSTAL AND RELEASE THE ENERGY/ENTITY

The client should accompany the healer to cleanse the crystal in the fire. First I ask my client if he is ready to let go of this energy/entity. Then I invite him to say goodbye to it in any way he needs, to thank it for the lessons it brought him, no matter how painful they have been. I build a fire right in my office in a brass bowl with Epsom salts and rubbing alcohol. I instruct my students to make sure that the metal bowl they use has no welds or seams on it, as the heat will rupture a seamed bowl. I have found that a seamless heavy-gauge aluminum bowl is good as well. I fill the bowl to a depth of about one inch with Epsom salts. Then I pour one ounce of rubbing alcohol into the bowl and light it carefully. This will produce a very hot fire that will burn for about three minutes. Do not add any more alcohol once the fire is burning, and wait until the fire is extinguished and the bowl has cooled off completely before relighting it. The flames from an alcohol fire are very hot and difficult to see in daylight. I dim the lights in my healing room to better see the flames when I pass the crystal through it. Be very careful as you perform this step, as you can easily get burned. Traditional healers use a bonfire, which is lit in a natural setting at night. They open sacred space, then call on the spirits who are in need of healing to come and warm their hands by the fire, and receive whatever care they need. The client is instructed to prepare a death arrow, a small stick on which she has symbolically carved or drawn the parts of herself that need to die—the character traits, symptoms, and behaviors that are no longer useful—which she prays over and then places into the fire. You can also build a conventional fire in your backyard or in a fireplace to clear a crystal. It's important that the crystal actually pass through the flames. I pass the crystal through the fire three times, then face South with the client by my side. I blow on the crystal to the South direction, then the West, the North, and the East. Afterward I cleanse the crystal with cold water. The intrusive energy/entity will feel the searing heat when you pass the quartz through the flames. The fire will expel the energy/entity from the crystal. This is the point when I perceive whether it is an energy or an entity. An entity will be received by luminous healers from the Spirit world who enter the safety of your sacred space. An intrusive energy will be combusted by the fire, its light and heat released to nature.

I once witnessed a jungle sorcerer extract an entity from a client and then hold the crystal very near the flames to make the entity suffer in the heat of the blaze. The sorcerer believed the entity had been sent by a rival sorcerer to harm his client, and he was intent on teaching it a scorching lesson. We do not do that. The flames are freeing the entity to return to the world of Spirit, where this being can finally achieve peace.

You will sometimes discover an intrusive entity hiding beneath an intrusive energy. After I complete the extraction and muscle test, my client should test strong. If she tests weak, I go back and track again. One such case happened with Therese.

Therese was a lay minister in a Catholic church in Cincinnati when she enrolled in the Healing the Light Body program. We decided to hold our final training session at the Canyon de Chelly National Park within the Navajo nation reservation. For many years Therese had felt slighted by the Church. Everyone recognized that she was the unifying force within her congregation. But since she was a woman in the Catholic faith, she had none of the rights and privileges of a priest to conduct religious ceremonies despite her comprehensive training in theology. According the Catholic dogma, she was permitted to address the congregation only as a prelude to the priest. She felt that she in particular and women in general were second-class citizens in the Church.

We were surrounded by thousand-foot-high red rock walls. Halfway up the cliff were the ruins of an ancient Anasazi dwelling. I had one student run energy along Therese's spine while two trackers monitored the location and movement of the intrusive energy. After a few moments of running energy along her spine, the trackers reported a dark mass ricocheting inside her Luminous Energy Field. It looked to them like a dark comet soaring inside her body. I held Therese's hands and closed my eyes so I could picture this energy. Slowly I began to draw out the energy through her fingertips and into the extraction crystal. It did not offer much resistance. The dark mass streamed into the crystal, where it was safely contained. The trackers reported the dark mass was gone. Then we retested Therese. During the Extraction she had reported no unusual feelings or sensations. Now she felt nauseous. To my surprise, she tested weak. She could barely hold her arm up in the air. I asked my assistant to run energy again. When I scanned Therese's Luminous Energy Field I perceived a man dressed in black garments like those Catholic priests wear. I felt a communication in my head, as if he were laughing and saying, She is mine, if you think you can take her, you've got a fight on your hands. It was as if I could hear these words inside my head and feel the hatred and bitterness in his tone.

An intrusive entity lay hiding underneath the energy we had extracted. I described what I had seen to Therese. She had a feeling that this man had made her life miserable sometime in the distant past. She saw herself punished for being a wise woman who had been perceived as a threat by the Church. This man had physically tortured her and made her suffering his personal cause, and his spirit continued tormenting Therese. Had he been in a body, he would have been magnetically drawn to Therese and become involved in her life in an equally destructive manner. In fact, she had manifested the same dilemma with the Church in this lifetime. She was still perceived as a threat. Today, of course, the instruments of torture are more subtle — shame, banishment, and disempowerment.

Here was a real "nasty." He believed that he possessed Therese and was sucking her life energy through her third chakra. It's not unusual for a parasitic entity to feel that it "owns" its host. He was intertwined along her spine, wrapping his tendrils of dark energy around the nerves extending from her spinal cord. His identity had become completely interwoven with hers.

Every intrusive entity is suffering and in need of healing. When I first learned the Extraction Process I would look forward to the occasional "nasty" entity. I considered it a test of my own skills. Now I have grown to understand that we have to love these entities, no matter how dark they appear to be. They, too, have come to us for healing. When we turn them over to the luminous healers in the Spirit world, they return gratitude and love to us, and on occasion will even return to assist us during a difficult Extraction.

I held Therese's hands and began to coax out the entity, speaking to him silently, letting him know that I was here to help end his suffering. The entity would have nothing of it. He laughed and scoffed at me. Meanwhile, Therese's knees buckled, and the tracker behind her had to support her weight. Her physical strength was gone, and she felt she was going to get sick at any moment. I asked the entity what it needed from Therese. He replied that he hated her and everything that she stood for—femininity, courage, and spirituality. I explained that he could find these qualities himself if he was receptive to healing. The entity laughed again. Then I began to feel the nausea. I was beginning to get dizzy and felt a metallic taste in my mouth. I asked Therese to count backward from twenty, and when she was halfway done I yanked the entity out. Therese collapsed to the ground. My nausea cleared immediately. I could feel the crystal get hot and start throbbing in my hand.

I passed the crystal around for the others to feel the energy within it. Everyone could sense the heat and intensity emanating from the quartz. After an Extraction the crystal must be held upright; be careful not to point either end toward you, since the energy-entity can sometimes escape and enter through one of your own chakras if you have an affinity for it, and then you will then need an Extraction performed on you. I caution students first learning this process that they may be unconsciously drawn to work with another student dealing with similar psychological issues, and the energy-entity can simply change hosts, leaving the client and lodging itself within the healer.

I handed the crystal to Therese, who was on the ground sobbing softly.

"This has been my battle all my life," she said. "I always thought I was born the wrong sex."

I asked Therese what she wanted to do with this entity.

"I feel like holding him over the fire and roasting him a little, to let him feel some of the pain he has been inflicting on me for so many years."

I asked Therese to carry the crystal for the next few days and to meditate on what it was she was receiving from this entity. There are always secondary benefits that an intrusive entity provides for a client. Sometimes it's a sense of purpose, or a cause to fight against, or a distorted mirror in which she can see her own reflection. Two days later Therese came to me and said she understood how this entity served her. He was the source of her anger toward the Church establishment, and in many ways toward the masculine. This anger had given her the strength to raise two daughters on her own and to emotionally support the women in her congregation. She was ready to forgive this entity and thank him for the valuable lessons she had learned. Had Therese attempted to heal herself through conventional psychotherapy, she would have arrived at many of the same insights. But insight does not equate to transformation. The intrusive entity would have remained comfortably lodged within Therese's Luminous Energy Field.

That evening we built a large fire. We called on the ancient dwellers of the canyons to come and be present in our ceremony. Then I asked Therese to accompany me to the fire and say goodbye to this being who had been with her for so long. She was ready to forgive him and set him free. I passed the crystal through the flames three times. When I blew the energy from the crystal into the South direction we felt a ball of light spring from the quartz. Everyone sensed the presence of heavenly spirits receiving this wounded soul. They held him tenderly, like a mother holding a child, and led him toward the light. Therese has since become a gifted healer in her own right. She has become known in her Christian community as a remarkable ceremonialist. She has left the established Church and is in high demand to perform weddings and other rites of passage.

CHAPTER 9

DEATH, DYING, AND BEYOND

The bus dropped us off at a spot where the dirt road crossed a dry riverbed. From here it was another two days on foot to the house of El Viejo, Antonio's teacher, now in his nineties. Somehow my mentor had gotten word that the old man was dying, and all of his students were gathering to honor his passing. Antonio had invited me to accompany him. I packed only the necessary gear: tent, sleeping bag, water filter, dried foods, and a camping stove, all stuffed into my backpack. Antonio smiled when he saw what I considered the "bare necessities" for this journey. He carried only his poncho and a small bag with quinoa, a grain domesticated by the Inka centuries ago. No pack, no sleeping bag. No load to shoulder.

We were the last to arrive. El Viejo lay in a fur-covered litter in the center of the room in the mud and stone hut. Candles were everywhere, and the scent of wax hung heavy in the air. The last rays of the sun filtered through the window, and by the half-light I could see the weathered brown faces of the men and women gathered here. All wore ponchos, some had shirts and sweaters, others hand-woven garments with the designs of their villages. All were in their fifties and sixties. One man, the youngest of the lot, played a bamboo flute in the corner. All had brought gifts for El Viejo—flowers, medicine stones, wooden keros, the ceremonial drinking vessels.

The old man was going to pass away that evening.

I sat in the corner next to the flute player and tried to make *myself invisible, but Antonio caught my eye and with a glance indicated I should join him by the old man. He held El Viejo's hand, and I could see in the old man's face a kindness and fearlessness I had never seen before. The old man nodded, and Antonio indicated I could return to my corner.*

One by one each of El Viejo's students kissed the old man. To each he gave a stone from his altar and a blessing. He gave Antonio a shiny object that I later discovered was a golden owl. Ancient. Pre-Columbian. Probably handed down from teacher to student for generations. Then he took a last, labored breath, and calm and peace came over his features. As he exhaled, my mentor pressed his lips to the old man's, received his final breath, and touched his lips to the woman next to him. In this way El Viejo's breath was exchanged from mouth to mouth around the room. Then someone opened the window, and the last person to receive the old man's breath released it toward the setting sun.

El Viejo was free.

JOURNALS

LIFE ENDS WITH THE LAST BREATH, JUST AS IT BEGINS WITH THE FIRST. Many of us grew up with the idea that when we died we would go to Heaven if we were good, but we would go to Hell if we were bad. The concepts of Heaven and Hell are strictly European. For the shaman there is no supernatural Heaven. Only the natural world exists, with its visible and invisible realms, among which is the Spirit world. Also, there is no independent evil principle in the Universe. Instead, we live in a benign Universe that takes a personal interest in our well-being. Evil exists only in the hearts of men and women. It is not a predatory outside force that we must guard against. When the missionaries began preaching about Hell, the Indians asked where it was located. The priests answered that it was not in the visible world. The closest analogy that they could imagine to describe the location of Hell was by pointing toward the ground below. This confused the indigenous Americans, for they understood that all life arises from the Earth.

As the physical body returns to the Earth, the soul prepares for its great journey home. When the brain shuts down, the electromagnetic field created by the central nervous system dissolves, and the Luminous Energy Field disengages from its former home. As this happens, the Luminous Energy Field grows into a translucent, egg-shaped torus that contains the other seven chakras, which continue to shimmer like points of light for the first few hours after death. If all proceeds smoothly, this luminous orb, which is the essence or soul of the individual, then travels through the axis of the luminous body, to become one with Spirit again. This occurs very quickly once the Luminous Energy Field is free from the body. The torus of the Luminous Energy Field squeezes through the portal created by its central axis, like a doughnut squeezing through its own hole.

When a dying person retains his awareness after death, he enters the light easily. My mentor compared this light to the dawn breaking on a cloudless morning, a state of primordial purity—immense and vast, defying description. The blackness of death, caused by the collapse of the senses, recedes and is dispelled by the light of Spirit.

The Huachipayre people of the upper Amazon believe that they can journey to the domains beyond death when they ingest *ayahuasca*, a hallucinogenic plant sacred to their people. During the ceremony they often experience terrifying visions of their death. In some cases they report being dismembered by a jaguar or swallowed by a gigantic anaconda. Once, while working with them, I felt my face pecked at by a gigantic eagle. Every time its beak tore into my flesh I would feel the piercing pain. Many of the initiatory rites of antiquity, including those of the Egyptians, Greeks, and Syrians, were designed to take the initiate through a similar process of symbolic death by which he ceased to identify with the mortal ego.

In my training with medicine people in the Amazon I experienced intricate death rites that stripped me of my ego self. During *ayahuasca* ceremonies I was terrified in ways I had never thought possible. Every demon imaginable appeared before me. My body was dismembered one hundred different ways. Then I was engulfed by white light and became inseparable from it. Over the years I returned many times to work with the *ayahuasca* shamans, and one day I discovered that I no longer needed to pass through fear in order to experience infinite light. That evening Don Antonio turned to me and said: "Death no longer lives within you. You have exorcised her from you. You can never be claimed by death."

My mentor prepared all of his life for this journey. Shortly before he died he explained to me how the steps of the journey were different for him as a shaman than for someone who was unprepared to meet his death. He fully expected to attain the freedom that is possible at the instant of death, during the dawning of the light of Spirit. At that moment, he explained, you perceive the dawn as if from the top of the world itself. You are taller than the highest mountains. Not only is the breaking dawn occurring outside you, but you simultaneously feel the sun rising in your belly and all of Creation stirring within you. You recognize that you are one with the dawning light. You surrender to the luminosity around you, are enfolded by it, and become one with it. During this stage you encounter luminous beings, medicine people who assist you in surrendering to the light. Inka legends say that we are all star travelers, and at this point in the dying process we can reembark on our great journey through the Milky Way.

If the person fails to recognize the dawn as the awakening of his own consciousness, the sun continues to rise in a million blinding, dazzling colors. All of nature comes alive in a stunning display of sound and light. It is as if the first day of Creation were replaying itself. In this stage, the forces of nature manifest in their pure essence. Already the one has separated into the many. Water appears as fluid light; the Earth appears as light; all of the elements are represented in their luminosity and coalesce into balls of energy. In this stage we have a second opportunity to recognize our luminous nature, to see that we are not separate from the dazzling light and energies around us. A shaman who has been preparing her entire life for this moment can attain liberation through the complete unfettering of consciousness during the first two stages of death. Others, however, may experience an instant of complete enlightenment, then slip back into unconsciousness. For them this process will go by in a flash of blinding light. They might not even realize they have passed through it.

The windstorm of death is so mighty that many people become unconscious and awaken only at the third stage of the journey. We observe that we still have a form, that we are a man or woman, that we can be young and unaffected by disease. But the dawn of consciousness has passed, and we are now in the twilight of the day. The colors are not as sharp or well defined, even though our awareness is tremendously heightened. Our ordinary senses are not separated from each other. We sense synesthetically with the totality of our being, and everything around us is alive. At this stage we go through our panoramic life review, in which every action, word, and deed we have performed appears before us and must be accounted for.

After the life review process we meet those who have died before us, including parents, friends, and people we may have hurt or wronged. My mentor explained to me that this domain has various levels, each one vibrating at a higher frequency than the one below it. The lower levels are very dense, associated with the domains of the Stone People and the Plant People. Persons trapped in these lower domains are undergoing purification in a world of darkness, where they have no eyes to see with or hands to feel with. They only sense the vague presence of others. These are Earth-bound domains for humans (although they are perfectly nice places for the Stone People). Here we relive our pain and suffering. The higher levels are joyful and filled with peace. We rejoin our loved ones and bask in the light of Spirit until our next incarnation. We naturally gravitate toward one level or another, depending on how we lived our life. We can see those in the levels below but cannot be seen by them, and we can speak and interact only with those in our level. The fourth level is our spiritual home, where we meet our ancestors and families.

The fifth world is the domain of luminous beings dedicated to assisting all humankind. Shamans who have mastered the journey beyond death return to this level. Long ago, when the shamanic death rites were first developed, this was a difficult level to attain. Today it is much more accessible. Trails have been blazed by the courageous men and women who have come before us. The prophecies of the Hopi and the Inka speak about our entire planet emerging into the fifth world. They refer to our entering the domains of angels. My mentor used to say to me, "We are here not only to grow corn, but to grow gods." I'm convinced that this is what he meant.

WHEN WE DIE

An extraordinary phenomenon occurs at the moment of death. When neural activity ceases and the brain shuts down, a portal opens between dimensions. The veils between the worlds part, enabling the dying person to enter into the world of Spirit. When a person has unfinished business in this world, she is unable to step easily through this portal. The biblical parable of the camel passing through the eye of a needle more easily than a rich man can enter heaven likewise addresses the difficulties met by those who have neglected the spiritual dimension in their pursuit of material gratification. We cannot carry our worldly identity into the beyond.

A person who is weighed down by heavy emotional baggage remains bound to the Earth. This soul has to go through a very intensive life review as soon as she arrives on the other side. Some people who have had a near-death experience recall a panoramic life review—a very detailed and comprehensive judgment day—even though the experience occurred in only minutes of Earth time. When the person does not return to the physical body, the life review can seem to take years, as the toxic energies in the Luminous Energy Field have to be combusted in an atmosphere where there is little air, which makes this clearing more difficult to accomplish.

After death, the Luminous Energy Field uncouples from the physical body. Two forces link the Luminous Energy Field to the body. The first is the electromagnetic field generated by the nervous system. When the field intensity drops to zero as the electrical activity in the brain ceases, the primary electromagnetic force that binds the luminous body to the physical body dissolves. The second link is the chakras, which secure the Luminous Energy Field to the spinal column. During the Final Rites we release every one of the seven bodily chakras, separate the luminous body from the physical, and seal the chakras so that the soul cannot reattach itself to the corpse again. When we disengage the chakras from the physical body we can return to the Earth what has always belonged to nature, and to the Heavens what has always belonged to Spirit.

On several occasions while training with my mentor I had the opportunity to visit a funeral home to observe the Luminous Energy Field of a deceased person. Every time I noticed that the luminous body remained connected at the belly to the corpse. Days later, when I visited the cemetery, I found the luminous body still hovering above the grave, attached to a decaying physical body that was no longer its home. Shortly before death, the doorway between the worlds opens. The shaman with whom I trained believed that forty hours after the last breath this portal shuts down. The soul then has to travel through all the planes where those who have not died consciously go to purge.

PREPARATION FOR PEACE

I feel that people should be allowed to die at home, where they are most comfortable and surrounded by a familiar environment. It is not as common nowadays for people to die at home. Most often death will occur in a hospital. Many doctors and nurses are as bewildered by death as the rest of us but may have become jaded by having to face death daily. Make sure that the hospital staff knows and respects the wishes of the dying person and her family. When the hospital staff has no explicit instructions from the dying person or next of kin, they must take whatever measures are necessary to prolong life. This legal mandate is designed to protect the hospital from potential lawsuits, and not to ensure the quality of life of the dying person or her family.

If your loved one is in a hospital, once you know there is nothing more that can be done medically, request a private room and have all monitors disconnected. Be sure that there are specific instructions in the chart that indicate her wish not to be resuscitated or have any extraordinary measures taken to revive her. Your written instructions and quiet fortitude will let the medical staff know that no heroics are necessary.

When the person is in the final stages of dying, request that all injections and invasive procedures be discontinued, except for medication to relieve pain. Invasive medical procedures can cause the dying person pain, anger, and confusion. If you are the next of kin, you have the authority to instruct the physicians to administer enough medication to alleviate pain but not so much that your loved one becomes unconscious.

People should be allowed to die in tranquility. A peaceful death is the most precious gift that we can offer a loved one. The person's senses are heightened, particularly her sense of hearing. Small noises can be painfully amplified and cause anxiety and confusion. Make this very difficult transition as gentle as possible. Your loved one's room should be a temple of peace at the time of her passing. Speak lovingly and frequently to her. If she is in a coma, and even after she has stopped breathing, the sound of your voice can be heard by her soul. Your love can reach her in dimensions you would never imagine.

Leave the body undisturbed for as long as possible after death. This

is very difficult to do in a hospital, but with some creativity and inge-
nuity you can secure at least a few hours of calm. The Luminous
Energy Field of the deceased undergoes tremendous flux when it disengages from the chakras. The luminous body expands in a whirl-
wind of energy and then contracts violently into the physical body,
yet cannot reanimate the body. In Tibet the body is watched over for
three days. Hospital regulations do not allow the body to remain without embalming for this length of time, which is another reason why
the procedures that follow are so important.

When my father died, I felt his luminous body float in the air for
two days until his funeral service, even though he was free from his
physical remains. My mother had organized a simple service at a
local church, and at the end of the ceremony I felt a breeze waft past
the altar; I sensed my father departing in a rush of light. When we
arrived at the cemetery an hour later the coffin felt devoid of any
energy.

DEATH RITES

I learned this technique from Doña Laura in the Andes. She was not
only a gifted midwife and shaman but also highly sought after for her
expertise in birthing people into the world of Spirit. Another student
of hers and I would assist her every opportunity we could. One time,
more than twenty years ago, I discovered how important these rites
were.

> The housekeeper had heard that someone had passed away, and
> Doña Laura sent Juan and me into town to practice seeing. This
> was my second such journey, and I did not look forward to the
> long ride into Cusco in a rattletrap bus along a dusty highway
> high in the Andes. The attendant at the funeraria, a boy in his
> late teens, was sweeping the mud that others had tracked in with
> them earlier in the day. It was nearly midnight, and there were

only two persons left from the service. Juan and I watched as the elder of the two women tossed the black shawl over her shoulders and gave the boy a coin on her way out the door.

I let Juan do the talking. After a few moments the boy led us into the room where the deceased lay in a simple wooden box inscribed with the Lord's Prayer. The boy nodded and closed the door. My companion removed three beeswax candles from his pack and set them around the wooden box. We walked back a half dozen paces, sat in our chairs, and practiced the Second Awareness exercise. No sooner had we started than Juan muffled a scream, scaring me half out of my chair. I have never enjoyed funerals, and I felt awkward at sneaking into one under the pretense of being distant relatives.

"Look," he said. I strained my eyes in the direction of the casket but could see only the flickering of the candles. "Look how it shimmers above the box!" Juan was easily excited, and I was beginning to get irritated, for I could see nothing. I stood up, walked close to the open wooden box, and looked in, expecting to see an old person, like the one we had seen in our previous visit. Instead, I saw an Indian girl no more than twelve years old; with rouge on her cheeks and a new red dress. The tears came streaming down my face. I knelt down on the pew beside the box and prayed for her as best I knew.

"Let's go," I said as I walked back toward Juan. Then I turned and saw the Luminous Energy Field, a golden orb hovering above the open box. The base of the orb was still connected to the physical body, somewhere between the heart and the belly. "Do you see that?" I asked Juan. "Claro," he said. Of course. "What are we going to do?" I asked. "Nothing," Juan replied. He reminded me that Antonio had made it clear that we were only to observe the departing luminous body and to say a prayer if we wished.

In a previous adventure, Juan and I had followed a recently deceased person to the cemetery and could see the luminous body literally sticking out of the earth, still attached to the physical one. Laura had explained to us that when a person dies unconsciously, he can remain trapped between the worlds, unaware that he has died, his luminous body still clinging to a lifeless physical form. A medicine person, she explained, would have helped him disengage from his physical body.

It took some pleading, but Juan agreed that we would attempt to set her free. Juan worked above the little body, disconnecting each of the chakras. I remained by the feet. After a few moments we stepped back and looked. The Luminous Energy Field was now an orb pulsing and glowing above the physical, almost with a heartbeat of its own. Juan and I nodded to each other, pleased. Her soul was free.

When we returned to our mentor's home we found him sitting at the dinner table, speaking softly with Doña Laura by the light of a candle. As soon as we entered the room they turned to us and asked us what we had done. "Nothing," we replied in unison. "Well, we had a cerveza, a beer, after we left the funeral home," I explained, knowing that Don Antonio was very strict about us not drinking. "That doesn't matter," he replied. And then Laura asked, "Who have you brought home with you?"

The soul of the young girl had followed us home. Antonio and Laura could see her hovering above us. While Juan and I had learned how to disengage the Luminous Energy Field from the physical body, we still had not learned the final rites. Antonio looked sternly at us and made us sit with Laura the remainder of the night while she assisted the girl in her journey back to infinity.

JOURNALS

The Death Rites help the dying person return to infinity. There are three steps to the Death Rites.

1. Recapitulation and forgiveness.
2. Granting permission to die.
3. The Final Rites.

RECAPITULATION AND FORGIVENESS

We want to assist a loved one in coming to closure with her life prior to death. It is as difficult to say "I forgive you" from the Spirit world and be heard by a living person as it is to say "I forgive you" to someone in a dream and have the real person hear you. When a person comes to closure with their worldly existence they transit effortlessly through the domains beyond death. Recapitulation and forgiveness bring completion to a life. Then, events from the past do not have to be forgiven during the life review that happens on the other side of life. The vast majority of reports in the literature on near-death experiences recount positive experiences. Yet cardiologist Maurice Rawlings interviewed individuals on the operating table immediately after they were resuscitated and found that nearly half of the people reported hellish encounters. Rawlings believes that many people have hellish visions that they repress in the days after resuscitation. Other researchers believe that these hellish visions may be self-inflicted. Raymond Moody, one of the foremost investigators of near-death experiences, states: "The judgment in the cases I studied came not from the being of light, who seemed to love and accept these people anyway, but rather from within the individual being judged." We are the accused, the defendant, the judge, and the jury all at once. How ready are we to forgive ourselves? Forgiveness and closure while we are still living is the focus of Recapitulation.

It is important for the family to give voice to the forgiveness and love that have not been expressed during the course of a lifetime. Atonement with the family is essential so that the person can pass on in peace. You would be surprised at the healing power of a simple "I love you" from a dying parent to a child or vice versa. This is not always easy, of course, yet a lifetime of mistakes can be undone through forgiveness even at the end of a life.

Recapitulation offers your loved one the opportunity to tell you her story. Having the opportunity to tell one's story has cathartic and healing power. It is the equivalent of doing your life review before you have actually died. Recapitulation is not a time for recriminations about past events. It is a time to listen to your loved one's story. The sooner you engage the Recapitulation and the more extensive the life review you accomplish, the easier the transition will be. Sometimes it is difficult to begin this conversation, especially if you have not had an intimate dialogue with your loved one in years. Find an entry point for dialogue. For example, ask your mother to recall the day she met your dad, how they courted each other, or what their first date was like. Engage her feelings by asking specific questions. What was her future husband wearing that day? Did she know he was the one when she met him? Be a good listener and ask questions. You will be surprised how readily a person will tell her story to someone who shows interest. Ask your loved one about her parents and her childhood. Where did she go to school? How did she dress? Whom did she have a crush on when she was in high school? What was her home life like? Gradually lead the conversation to more personal topics: Whom does she need to forgive? Remind your loved one that she can forgive anyone through a prayer or a blessing. Ultimately, the dying person needs to forgive herself and know that she is fully forgiven by life. Lastly, ask her how she would like to be remembered. What are the stories she would like her grandchildren to remember her by? Recapitulation brings closure through forgiveness. Assist your loved one to let go of any feelings of having been wronged or having wronged anyone else.

In the weeks before my father passed away, we sat together every day while he told me the story of his life. At the beginning he was hesitant, but soon he was flooded with images from his past. It was as if a dam had broken, and reflections and feeling flowed freely. It began with an exercise in guided imagery in which we envisioned ourselves sitting on a large boulder beside a river. He described the images that he saw floating down the river. At first the water was gray and murky. Then after a few days scenes from his childhood drifted by, and he described these to me as if he were seeing them in a dream. Sometimes he sobbed quietly. Later he told me about a man whom he had wronged during his adolescence but whom he hadn't thought about in decades. I encouraged him to feel forgiven and to forgive this man in return. Lastly, images of my mother and their children appeared. He recounted all of this in great detail before dozing off tranquilly. This was a private process shared only by the two of us, yet at the end he was able to call our family together and tell each one of us how much he loved us. This was the first time any of us had heard him say "I love you." He had wanted to express this all his life but had never been able to bring himself to do so before.

Tremendous forgiveness can occur in the Recapitulation. But do not expect to be a miracle worker and think that you can achieve in a few hours the healing that could not be accomplished in a lifetime. People tend to die in the same way that they have lived. It's natural for your loved one to experience anger when faced with the end of his life, and you can easily become the target of his resentment. Be careful not to react to it or to take it personally. Powerful realizations often come uninvited as one approaches death. One of them is understanding that we could have lived differently, loved more fully, and forgiven more readily. This anger is not being directed toward you personally. Make it okay for your loved one to voice his feelings, and respond to his anger with physical comfort and support. Hold your loved one's hand as he cries or expresses his ire. Be an unshakable source of love and unconditional support even in a storm of rage. The more willing your loved one is to forgive himself, the more quickly his rage will turn into compassion.

If your loved one's condition is critical and he has not been informed of this, by all means let him know. Most people know anyway. They can feel the change in attitude among the family members present—the new quietness in the room, the hushed voices, the forced smiles. It is best to be direct, yet gentle and compassionate. Your straightforwardness will give your loved one permission to be open and disclosing with you. He will know that he can count on you to speak the truth.

GRANTING PERMISSION TO DIE

Perhaps the most important step in the Death Rites is giving a loved one permission to die. Let them know that there is no reason to worry about those who stay behind. A student of mine named Diane sat beside her dying mother for weeks. The older woman was unable to let go, despite the fact that she was in a great deal of pain and could no longer eat. Diane had performed several Illuminations on her mother, and she and her sister had begun to forgive each other and heal the lesions of the past. It finally occurred to Diane that she and her sister had not let their mother know that it was all right for her to leave. She finally said, "Mother, we are here with you and love you very much. We want you to know that we will be okay. We will look after each other and keep our family together. Even though we will miss you, it is perfectly natural for you to go. We will treasure all of the beautiful moments that we had together, but we don't want you to suffer anymore, or to continue to cling to life. You have our full and complete permission to die. You know that we will always love you." A few hours later her mother took her final breath and died peacefully.

Without your permission to die, your loved one might cling to life for months, enduring unnecessary suffering and causing great anguish for the family. Permission must come from the immediate family, and ideally there should be a consensus. If there is a dissenting family member who won't let go, encourage him to express his love and forgiveness nonetheless. I have observed that the family members who have the hardest time letting go are the ones who have the most unfinished business with the dying person or who are the most frightened of their own death. Every voice in the room must count and be heard. If you are working with a client, make sure that all immediate relatives voice their feelings to the dying person. As the healer, you can add your consent as well, but remember that permission from those closest to the client carries the most weight, even if this happens to be a personal friend and confidant and not an immediate family member.

THE FINAL RITES

You do not need to be a shaman or a priest to perform the Final Rites. You can hold the space for a loved one to be touched by the hand of Spirit. There are two parts to the Final Rites: the Illumination Process and the release of the Luminous Energy Field. I've had many clients tell me that they've felt the presence of their deceased relatives as well as luminous beings around them during the Illumination Process. It's as if spiritual midwives on the other side are preparing to receive the dying person.

Through the Illumination Process you can create the space where a loved one can experience grace and liberation. It is easy to feel overwhelmed by the idea that you must accomplish a lifetime of healing in a few days. It is even more overwhelming if the loved one is close to dying. Remember, though, that it is never too late for healing. With the immediacy of death comes the realization that we have no time to waste. There is no tomorrow in which to attend to the healing we have put off all our lives. A friend who is a Roman Catholic priest once commented to me that the confession a dying person makes is the most important one, because it is the most sincere. You will find this healing to be one of your most powerful life experiences.

It is best to begin the Illumination Process some time before your loved one passes, as it can require several sessions to clear the toxic energy around a lifetime of imprints. Do not be afraid that you will pick up any toxic residues adhering to the person's chakras, as these are combusted and turned into light. You are in no jeopardy whatsoever. The process happens at an energetic level and not psychologically, so these energies do not surface as anger and resentments.

Should you find that a loved one's religious beliefs do not allow her to experience an Illumination, do not force it upon her. You are not there to convert anyone to your beliefs. You are there to help the person find the strength, guidance, and spiritual fortitude to embark on the greatest journey of her life. I remember attending a friend's father, a very religious man in his early eighties. When my friend explained the healing work that I did, his father stared at him in disbelief. The old man thanked his son but let him know that his priest came by his hospital room every morning to pray with him, and that this was enough. The father was well traveled, and we struck up a conversation about the Peruvian rain forest, which he had visited as a young man. We began to exchange stories about river ports in the Amazon. He would doze off after a few minutes of conversation. On my third visit I asked him if he would mind if I prayed with him. He indicated that it would be fine, and I took his hand and closed my eyes in prayer. I had noticed that his wife was the only person who touched him; all the children kept their distance, even while taking part in animated conversations. It was as if they were afraid that dying might be contagious and did not want to risk infection through physical contact. Every time we closed our eyes to pray he would grasp my hand and be asleep within minutes.

It is essential that you obtain your loved one's permission before you perform an Illumination or any part of the Death Rites. My friend's father had given me permission to pray with him. This was all I needed to perform an Illumination. It was very awkward to reach behind his head to hold the deepening and release points, as the hospital bed was against a wall. I performed the Illumination by his side, simply holding his hand, silently asking his body-mind to activate the deepening points every time I pressed a point in his hand and to activate the release points every time I pressed a different point. My client was ready to take part in the healing. His body-mind readily complied, making the necessary luminous connection between the points in the hand and the back of the head.

The points I work with on the wrist are on the same acupuncture meridians as the deepening and release points. The deepening points in the hand are located on the outside of the wrist, on the wrinkle of the wrist joint. The release points are located about one inch above the wrist, on the top and bottom of the forearm. I opened the chakra we were working on and closed it when we were finished. In three sessions we completed Illuminating all seven chakras. My friend's father would wake up after each Illumination and tell me how restfully he had slept, or how he had dreamed. I taught my friend how to perform the Final Rites on his father because I was going to be away. On my return I learned that he had passed away during his sleep.

The Illumination Process combusts the energy in the chakras and erases imprints from the Luminous Energy Field. This alleviates the life review process in the Spirit world, as most of the charge has been drained from emotional memories. Since you will be Illuminating all seven chakras, you do not need to test for a compromised chakra. When you've cleared the sludge from the first chakra, balance it by spinning it clockwise again, and proceed to the second chakra, following the protocol in the Illumination Process. You will probably not be able to Illuminate all seven chakras in one session — the process can be lengthy.

The body knows how to die in the same way that it knows how to be born. Nine out of ten times the Luminous Energy Field returns to the world of Spirit with ease. Similarly, nine out of ten births happen without complications. During childbirth, one in ten is not an

THE SPIRAL OF CHAKRAS FOR THE FINAL RITES

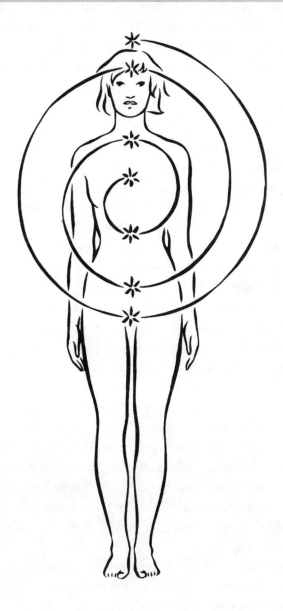

acceptable level of risk, and even natural births are generally planned to take place in a hospital within easy reach of a physician. The disengaging of the chakras during the Final Rites is necessary only when the process does not happen naturally. These are the rites you will perform after the person has died. You release the Luminous Energy Field and seal the chakras immediately after death so that the luminous body does not reenter the physical shell or become contaminated by the energy residues in the body.

1. **Open sacred space, calling in the four directions, Heaven, and Earth** (see Chapter 6).

2. **Expand your luminous body over yourself and your loved one.** It is important to work within this doubly sacred space. The sacred space protects your loved one from disruptive outside energies. The legends of the rain forest peoples say that at the moment of death the hungry ghosts of all those whom we have hurt or offended gather around our deathbed to claim their due. They follow the deceased until they have achieved retribution. I prefer to interpret these hungry ghosts as psychological demons representing all of the unfinished business from our past. That's why it is so important to reach closure with our life. Once we do so, the hungry ghosts are dispelled; forgiveness dissolves them into thin air. When you expand your luminous field over your loved one, you are creating an island of tranquility in the middle of a storm. In this island, relatives who have passed on and healers from the Spirit world assist the dying person. There is a saying among the shamans of the upper Amazon that the purpose of all of their training is to learn how to leave this life alive. This doesn't mean that they intend to take their physical bodies with them, but that they seek to maintain their consciousness intact through the journey.

3. **After your loved one stops breathing, disengage the chakras.** Ideally this step should be performed immediately after the person passes, and in any case no later than forty hours after the final breath. Immediately after death the chakras begin to release the luminous

threads that once connected them to events from the past. The rhythm of the chakras changes. One can feel the frequency and vibration of each chakra increase. They begin to disengage from the body but are hampered by the sludge within them.

Because the energy of the chakras is changing very rapidly, we disengage them following the arc of a spiral, with the heart at the center. Each chakra must be spun counterclockwise. Place your hand over your loved one's heart chakra, then spin your fingers counterclockwise three or four times to unwind this center. Continue to the solar plexus, then the throat, next the second chakra, then the sixth, next the root chakra, and last the crown in the steps described below. As you unwind the chakras, imagine that you are making a great spiral with the heart as its center. Follow these steps carefully.

4. Draw an arc of a spiral with your hand as you move to the third chakra or solar plexus, repeating the procedure above. When you have unwound the third chakra, go back to the heart, feel that chakra, and retrace the arc of a spiral down to the third and up to the throat chakra.

5. Repeat with each chakra, returning to the heart after you disengage each energy center. The last chakra that you release will be the crown. By this time you will have drawn a great spiral over the person's body multiple times. Your loved one's luminous body may exit through any one of the seven chakras.

6. Push energy through your loved one's feet to "nudge" the luminous body free. Place the palms of your hands on the soles of your loved one's feet, so that your right palm is resting on his left sole, and vice versa. Visualize energy gushing out of your hands into his body. The Luminous Energy Field sometimes adheres to the chakras even after they have been unwound. This step nudges the Luminous Energy Field so it breaks free from the body. In most cases the luminous body exits immediately after the chakras have been disengaged, and it becomes unnecessary to perform this step or the next.

7. Draw out the luminous body. Move to the person's head and cradle it in your hands. Hold the head gently for a few moments, letting her know that it's okay for her to let go. Tell her that you will be fine and that you love her. Remember that she can still hear you. Speak these words softly yet firmly. Draw your hands back, exerting gentle pressure on her head, and draw out her luminous body through the crown chakra. You will feel a tremendous surge of energy as the Luminous Energy Field becomes free of the body. One student reported that he and his siblings went from despair to joyful tears when their mother's luminous body became free. The entire room was filled with a peace that they could not explain. The luminous body may not always exit through the crown. It will exit through whichever chakra it is most ready to depart from. I have seen cases in which the luminous body has departed through the second chakra or the heart chakra.

8. Seal the chakras by making the sign of a cross over each center with your thumb. Sealing the chakras keeps the luminous body from returning to a lifeless physical form. You can use holy water or an essential oil for this. Remember that the cross is more ancient than Christianity. It represents the sealing of a doorway into a physical body that will never be used again.

In the Christian traditions one finds a similar practice associated with the last rites, except that the meaning of these rites has largely been forgotten. The priest anoints the forehead and heart, making the sign of the cross on them with holy water. He is likely to be unaware that he may be trapping the person's Luminous Energy Field within the physical body, binding spirit to matter in a lifeless shell. When this happens a person can continue identifying with a decaying physical body. If he is the one in ten who did not return to the Spirit world naturally, he may not be free until the body completely decomposes and there is no matter left for the luminous body to adhere to.

The first time I administered the Death Rites, outside of assisting my mentor, was when my father died. I was with him when he entered into a coma. My sister, my mother, and I kept vigil by his bedside, holding his hand for days and letting him know he was loved, that we would be okay, that he need not worry about us. At the end of one of these sessions my sister and I stepped out to get a sandwich. On our return we saw that he had stopped breathing. A young Roman Catholic priest was standing over the bed administering the last rites. I gently nudged the priest out of the room and locked the door. As I disengaged my father's chakras, I observed his luminous body exit through his heart. As soon as his chakras were free, his luminous body broke free from the physical. All it took was a nudge of love through the soles of his feet. The quality of the room changed. We felt a serenity that I associate with cathedrals more than with hospitals. My mother stopped crying and the three of us hugged each other. We sensed my father's presence in the room and felt that he was free from the crippling pain he had been in for the last year. I sealed his chakras, opened the door, and invited the young priest to complete his ceremony.

SPIRITUAL ASSISTANCE

The healer must render spiritual assistance to the dying in as unobtrusive a manner as possible. Keep in mind that everyone around you is in need of healing, not just the dying person. Sometimes the family will want you to assume the leading role simply to avoid dealing with death. Be careful not to become caught in this predicament. The most important task of the healer is to hold sacred space. During the dying process every feeling is amplified. Painful events from the past, the confusion of dying, and the grief of family members in the room all add to the chaos. When you hold a loved one within your Luminous Energy Field, you are creating an oasis of peace. In that calm it is possible for the dying person to regroup, rec-

ognize loved ones, and discover the luminous healers awaiting on the
other side.

SYMBOLIC DEATH

Shamans learn the journey beyond death through the Spirit Flight.
They believe that it is important to learn the path to infinity now,
while we still have a body to which we can return. They engage in
rituals in which they symbolically die and journey to the world
beyond death, where they receive powerful healing gifts. By practicing the Spirit Flight (sometimes called an out-of-body experience in
the West) and meditation, the medicine person learns the maps to the
afterlife. On the other side of life they discover only life. The journey
beyond death has become an archetypal symbol of transformation
and is found in every culture in the world. This journey into a divine
reality is illustrated by Christ, who spent three days among the dead
before reappearing on Earth.

The oral traditions of indigenous people abound with stories
describing the challenges one might face in the journey toward the
light. These tests include meeting demonic figures, multiheaded
monsters, ghouls, ghosts, and specters—in short, all the characters of
a really bad nightmare. Mythology provides us not only with detailed
descriptions of these encounters, but also the strategies used to conquer them. If you study the stories carefully, you discover that the
hero achieves success by shifting her awareness and not through battle. When Hercules faced the many-headed serpent Hydra, he discovered that every time he cut off one head, two more would grow.
One Amazon shaman told me of when he encountered a gigantic
anaconda during a Spirit Flight journey. No matter how fast he ran,
the serpent kept gaining on him. Finally it reared before him and
opened its cavernous maw. He saw the ribbed palate at the roof of its
mouth and was certain the serpent would devour him. At that point,
trembling with fear, he jumped down the anaconda's throat and was

swallowed by the great animal. His body was squeezed until all of his bones were crushed. Then he found that he was able to see through the serpent's eyes and feel the texture of the ground under his belly. He completed his journey in the shape of that great snake, and now the serpent guides him every time he embarks on the Spirit Flight.

Every religion has a body of work describing the journey beyond death, with instructions on how to attain liberation and details of what we will find when we get there. The best known are the writings found in the Tibetan Book of the Dead, which, like its Egyptian counterpart, was prized not only for its maps of the Spirit world but because it revealed the secret of life. The maps are useful in death, but they are more important to help us understand the mystery of being alive. Once we understand the continuity of life throughout eternity we attain freedom. Death ceases to stalk us, and we discover a self that dwells in infinity.

EPILOGUE

MACHU PICCHU WAS BUILT BY PACHACUTEK, THE NINTH INKA KING, who ruled an empire the size of the United States. His name means "renewer of the world" and embodies the essence of the Inka prophecies that herald the period of renewal at the end of time, or *pachacuti*. The word *pacha* in the language of the Inka means "Earth" or "time." *Cuti* means "to turn upside-down." *Pachacuti* therefore refers to a time of great upheaval on the Earth. The last *pachacuti* happened with the arrival of the Spanish conquistadors, when the Indian world was turned upside-down and order was replaced with chaos. Kings and chiefs were put to death, medicine people were enslaved, and Indians were worked ruthlessly in plantations and mines. The next *pachacuti*, according to the Inka shamans, has already begun, and the upheaval and chaos characteristic of this period will last until the year 2012. During this time the world will be turned right side up again. The paradigm of looting and pillaging the Earth brought by European civilization will end, and the ways of the Earth peoples will make a comeback. The conquistador will perish by his own blade. The Earth will return to balance.

For the Inka this *pachacuti* means the end of the world as we know it. Although the prophecies mention the possibility of annihilation, they actually promise the dawn of a millennium of peace, beginning after this period of turmoil. Even more important for the shamans, the prophecies speak about a tear in the fabric of time itself, a window into the future through which a new human species will emerge. Don Antonio used to say that *Homo sapiens* has perished, and that a new human, *Homo luminus,* is being born this very instant on our planet. Interestingly, my mentor believed that evolution happens within generations, not in between generations, as biology believes. This means that *we* are that new human. We are the ones that we've been waiting for. Our question no longer is can we make a quantum leap into who we are becoming, but rather dare we do so.

Don Manuel Quispe had achieved a truly global perspective. He understood that the destinies of the peoples of the Earth are all inter-woven. He believed the Inka prophecies, like those of the Hopi and the Maya, were for peoples of all colors and nations. They were founded on *munay,* the unqualified power of love.

Over the years Don Manuel welcomed me into his most pri-vate ceremonies. I recall meeting the eldest of the Inka medi-cine men, the equivalent of the Dalai Lama, during a ceremony outside Cusco. We were sitting in an Inka ruin, surrounded by mountain peaks that towered more than a mile above us even though we were already at an altitude of eleven thousand feet. The shaman held three coca leaves between his fingers and began to pray. He blew his prayers onto the leaves and called on the spirit of the mountains and of Mother Earth. I felt as if the snow-capped peaks were present in our ceremony. Suddenly they weren't around and above me, but next to me, or perhaps I was next to them, in the green valleys in between. He believed that the healing ceremonies and the knowledge of the Indios belonged to the entire planet. This was made clear to me during an expedition to the holy mountain, Ausangate.

We were at Pachanta Pampa, preparing for the final leg of the journey to our camp at fourteen thousand feet. For the next six days I would live, eat, and take part in ceremony with the Inka elders. Mt. Ausangate is nearly twenty-two thousand feet above sea level and is known as the "mountain enshrouded in storm." We were making our ascent in July, the middle of winter in South America. According to legend, the clouds that continually envelop the mountain part when shamans come for ceremony at the *huaca*, a place of power right at the heart of the mountain.

"You have to bring the blindfold down over the horse's eyes before you mount him," the Indian man explained in a mixture of Spanish and Q'echua. "He spooks easily." I looked at my horse, barely larger than a pony, and the bandana that covered his eyes, and muttered, "Damn," under my breath. "He's a good horse," the Indian went on, noticing my hesitation. "Small but good. Big horses, their hearts give out at this altitude." I looked up, and there wasn't a patch of blue in the sky. In fact, it looked as though it would begin snowing at any moment. This didn't seem like my day. I turned to the man holding my blindfolded horse and said, "I think I'll walk. *Muchas gracias.*"

Huacas are holy, but they are also dangerous places, where the veil between the worlds thins, where ordinary perceptions of time and space blur. They are places where the *causay*, the original energy of Creation, seeps into our world, where shamans can influence events that occurred in the past, and where they can read destiny. The most powerful of all the Inka *huacas* is on Mt. Ausangate. Every year seventy thousand pilgrims, many of them medicine men and women, meet at the mountain for the largest Indian celebration in the Americas, Collor R'iti, the Feast of the Snow Star. The festivity is held in the "public" part of the mountain. We were going into the heart of the mountain, to a location at the foot of the glacier known only to Don Manuel and the other elders. We were coming to witness the reading of the Inka prophecies of the time to come.

At fourteen thousand feet, every step up is a meditation. Three hours into our trek I regretted not having taken a horse, blindfolded or not. The unexpected blessing was that I got to walk with the party of more than fifty shamans. On my side was Don Manuel. He explained that Inka don't ride horses. "They are Spanish," he had said. The remaining members of our group had taken a longer trail, better suited for horses. We were taking a footpath that required us to wade through knee-high glacial streams. My Gore-Tex boots were soaked through, and as I squished with every step the women laughed and pointed out how much better their sandals made from old rubber tires were. They dried quickly in the thin air.

"We've lived in the mountains since the beginning of time," Don Manuel explained, "even before the founding of the city of Cusco. After the Ñaupa Runa, the preworldly beings, were banished by the Children of the Sun, our ancestors settled in the mountaintops. We've always lived with the *apus*, the sacred mountains." At the time of the Spanish conquest a group of Inka shamans returned to the mountaintops to escape the Church and the conquistadors. For centuries they were thought to be the stuff of legend, a myth from the distant past. Then nearly fifty years ago they came down from the mountaintops for the feast of Collor R'iti and were recognized by the medicine peoples as the last of the Children of the Sun. Legend has it that when they first appeared wearing their ponchos with the royal emblem of the Sun, an aisle parted down the middle of the thousands gathered, and the elders welcomed them, saying: "We have been waiting for you for five hundred years."

When I asked Don Manuel why they came down from their high mountains, he said that it had been foretold in their prophecies. For five hundred years they have watched the working of the conquistadors—the polluting of the rivers, the building of the cities, the changing weather patterns, and other signs. He explained that they had been entrusted with a prophecy that announced the end of time. "Anyone can be a soothsayer," Don Manuel explained. "We have been the keepers of a body of processes, of rites, that usher in who we are becoming as a people, as a planet. These processes are not only for the Indians, but for the entire world. It is known as the *mosok karpay*, the rites of the time to come."

I asked Don Manuel to explain what these processes were. "Our prophecies are written in stone," he said. "We have no written language, like you do. We have only our weavings and our stones. If you understand Machu Picchu and the stones at that ancient city," he went on, "you understand Cusco. Machu Picchu is a miniature of Cusco. If you understand Cusco, you understand the entire Inka empire." At that point he paused, and I seized the opportunity to lean against a boulder to catch my breath. We were within one mile of Azulcocha, our base camp at the Blue Lagoon at the heart of the mountain. All around us were *apachetas*, piles of prayer stones built by pilgrims who had undertaken the same journey we were embarked upon. The stones had been carefully laid one upon the other, making towers five to six feet high. The boulder I was leaning on had one of these *apachetas* on it, and Don Manuel pointed out that they marked the entry into the inner space, the heart of the mountain. Don Manuel squatted down next to me and opened his *mesa*, the collection of stones and power objects that every shaman carries. "If you understand the *mesa*," he said as he carefully unfolded his medicine bundle to reveal the rocks inside, "you understand Machu Picchu and the prophecies."

The shaman earns her *mesa* during the course of her own healing. Each stone represents a wound that has been transformed into a source of wisdom and courage. In the process she clears the karmic imprints in her Luminous Energy Field and the toxic sludge that blemishes her chakras. Being free of the grip of past imprints, she can be informed by who she is becoming. Her chakras extend luminous strands that span the fabric of time and anchor themselves to infinity. Through these fibers of light the wisdom and teachings of time past and future flow. She remembers the ancient stories and recalls the ones that have not been yet told. And she can grow a body that ages, heals, and dies differently. She can become an Inka, a child of the sun, *Homo luminus*.

> *The end of the tyranny of time...every religion in the world speaks to it. In Judaism the Messiah will come at the end of time. In Christianity, time ended once with the coming of Christ, and then again at the end of time when "the living and the dead shall*

238 / ALBERTO VILLOLDO

rise and be judged." Interesting how they all assume that time flows in one direction only, that the end of time is something that will happen when we run out of minutes and seconds.

I've discovered that for Antonio, Laura, Manuel, and their cohorts, stepping outside of time is a process, not something that will happen in some distant future. Its key ingredient is the Illumination Process. Instead of holding a sacred space open for a few moments and bringing the causay energy for healing, they enter into the space, return to the source they call the texemuyo. My Jesuit priest friend has been nagging me to bring him to this ceremony, but I refuse to. In it the shaman retrieves that self that never left the Garden of Eden, that still speaks with God, that does not die. Pretty heady stuff. Everyone else is waiting for eternity, and the shamans are saying, "How about tonight?"

The problem with time as we know it is that it is wedded to causality. Cause and effect. Who I am today is the result of what happened yesterday or ten years ago. Among the curses that come with causality are psychologists. They pick at the weeds that were seeded during childhood, raking up their leaves and cutting off their stems, but never pulling up the roots. They continue harvesting pathology and forget to plant the seeds of future possibility. Causality condemns you to the ordinary and the commonplace.

I'm interested in this idea of noncausal relationships. Antonio says that he was the one who orchestrated our meeting. It would have been impossible to find him by looking, he claimed. If five hundred years of conquistadors and missionaries had not found him and his people, who was I to think I could have done so?

Tonight is a good night to step outside of time. Infinity is patient.

JOURNALS

INDEX

I invite you to let me know of your experiences with the shamanic healing processes. Send an e-mail to Dr. Alberto Villoldo, villoldo@thefourwinds.com. I would love to hear about your successes and stories. You can also visit our Web site, thefourwinds.com, for additional articles, photographs, and video clips of the shaman healers.

For information on Healing the Light Body School and training programs offered by Dr. Alberto Villoldo, please visit our Web site or call (310) 454-0444.